Detoxification Made Simple

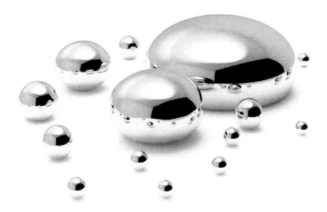

The fast-track to becoming a less stressed,

more energized, healthier version of you!

Table of Contents

Introduction 9

Disclaimer 13

Chapter 1: METALS IN THE HOME 15
    LEAD 17
    CADMIUM 21
    ALUMINUM 22
    MERCURY 24
    ELEMENTAL MERCURY 25
    INORGANIC MERCURY 26
    ORGANIC MERCURY 27
    ARSENIC 29

Chapter 2: WHEN HEAVY METALS BECOME KRYPTONITE 33
    THE PITUITARY GLAND 37
    SLEEP 38
    THE WEAKEST LINK 39
    WHEN SILVER BECOMES MERCURY 40
    FURTHER DISRUPTION 42
    ZINC AND COPPER 43
    BRAIN FOG AND FATIGUE 44

Chapter 3: TESTING FOR HEAVY METALS 47
- THE HAIR ANALYSIS TEST 49
- CHALLENGE TEST (URINE) 50
- BLOOD TEST 52
- THE IMPORTANCE OF TRI-TESTING. 53
- DON'T BE GREEDY 54

Chapter 4: DETOXIFICATION PATHWAYS 55
- LUNGS 56
- HELP FOR POORLY FUNCTIONING LUNGS 58
- SKIN 59
- HELP FOR YOUR SKIN 60
- KIDNEYS 61
- HELP FOR YOUR KIDNEYS 63
- THE LYMPHATIC SYSTEM 64
- HELP FOR YOUR LYMPHATIC SYSTEM .. 65
- THE DIGESTIVE SYSTEM 66
- HELP FOR YOUR DIGESTIVE SYSTEM 68
- THE LIVER 69
- IT'S ALSO A GIVER 70
- WAYS TO HELP YOUR LIVER 72

Chapter 5: THE MISSING LINK - SLEEP 75
- TICK-TOCK 77
- MAGNESIUM 81
- SALT AND SODA BATHS 81
- SPIKE LAVENDER 82
- CBD OIL 83

BETA-1, 3D GLUCAN 84

Chapter 6: PRE-TOX BEFORE YOU DETOX 87
BLOCKED PATHWAY TEST 89
THE 5'p.S. OF PREPARATION 90
PHYSICAL STRESS..91
EMOTIONAL STRESS 93
CHEMICAL STRESS..94
REMINERALIZE 95
SELENIUM..97
BEET JUICE IS HARD TO BEAT 98
WHY BROCCOLI IS A SUPER SPROUT. 99

Chapter 7: IT TAKES GUTS TO LEAK 101
GLUTEN-FREE? - Not so fast. 105
S.O.S … I STILL NEED TO FIX MY GUT ..107

Chapter 8: STOMACH ACID IS STRONG FOR A REASON 109
HEARTBURN—A BILLION DOLLAR INDUSTRY 111
NOW IT GETS TRICKY 115
RECAP 116
STOMACH ACID TEST 117
HOW TO FIX LOW STOMACH ACID........118

Chapter 9: OPENING CLOSED DETOX DOORS 121
WHY STRESS MAKES A MESS....................124
DRAINAGE AND BILE 126

Chapter: 10: BURLY BINDERS 133
- #1 ACTIVATED CHARCOAL 135
- #2 BENTONITE CLAY 139
- #3 CHLORELLA 139
- BLENDING OUR ABC's 140
- #4 MODIFIED CITRUS PECTIN 141
- #5 IMD (Intestinal Metal Detox) 142
- #6 ZEOLITES 143

Chapter 11: DETOXIFICATION UNLEASHED 145
- GLUTATHIONE 146
- Nrf2 149
- SULFORAPHANE 155
- SUPPLEMENTS 156
- PULSING 157
- FASTING 159
- INFRARED 160

MORE BOOKS BY THIS AUTHOR 166

WHAT AM I UP TO NOW? 167

NEWSLETTER DETAILS 168

SEE YOUR NAME IN PRINT 169

SAUNA DISCOUNT CODE 170

Copyright 2019 ©

No part of this book is to be copied, republished, or reproduced without written permission from the author. Requests made can be made through the James Lilley Facebook page. You can also stay in my loop via my newsletter at
https://www.writeonjames.com/

Introduction

Hello, and thank you for taking the time to open this book. Heavy metals are a topic I am passionate about. Over the years, I've spent hundreds of hours listening to lectures on the subject. I've also spent a great deal of time reading the latest literature. But more importantly, I understand the devastation they cause on a personal level.

Rest assured, this book contains everything you need to get your health on track. Inside, we'll cover what heavy metals are, how they get inside us, and what you can do to remove them from your body. The entire detoxification process has been mapped out, step-by-step. This information is easy to follow and enjoyable to read.

Some of these detoxification techniques may require the assistance of a healthcare provider, while others you can do from home. That said, this book is *not* intended to treat or diagnose any illness. What follows is intended for informational purposes only. At this point, you may be asking if this book has anything of value to offer. That's a fair question, and it's worthy of an honest answer.

Sudden exposure to certain toxic metals may require a hurried visit to your local ER. Chances are, the staff treating you will save your life. Doctors and nurses perform such medical miracles every second of every day. They deserve our utmost respect, and we can learn a lot from them. **But not all exposure to heavy metals is sudden or obvious.**

Often, the road to illness can be slow and meandering. Symptoms of fatigue, brain fog, depression, and anxiety can affect our bodies for years without anyone making a connection to heavy metals toxicity. In short, there are times when heavy metals fail to show up on a busy doctor's radar. And yet, they are inextricably linked to many forms of illness.

It doesn't matter what your doctor calls it, it ALWAYS involves toxicity—Dr. Sherry Rogers

In 1974, the World Health Organization (WHO) went as far to report that 82% of all chronic degenerative disease was caused by toxic metal poisoning. Since then, heavy metals have continued to be an insidious part of our lives. They find their way into our food, our water, and even the air we breathe. And while heavy metals are obviously a cause for concern, there's also some good news!

Your body has six main detoxification pathways, each are covered in this book. With the right approach, these pathways can be optimized leading to a level of health you may not have experienced before. This becomes the turning point for a less stressed, more energized, healthier version of you.

We have a lot of ground to cover, and I'm excited to share my understanding of heavy metals with you. I know what it's like to crave *simple* solutions, and I'll attempt to convey this message in the least complicated way. You might want to grab a pen and paper to take notes along the way.

Without further ado, let's get started!

Disclaimer

Every effort has been made to ensure that the information contained in this book is complete and accurate. The statements made in this book have not been evaluated by the US Food and Drug Administration (FDA.) The products mentioned in this book are not intended to treat, diagnose, cure, or prevent any disease. The information provided in this book is not a substitute for a consultation with your own physician and should not be construed as individual medical advice.

Although this book contains information relating to health care, the information is not intended as medical advice and is not intended to replace a person-to-person relationship with a qualified healthcare professional. If you know or suspect you have a health problem, it is recommended that you first seek the advice of a physician before trying out any medical program or treatment. All efforts have been made to assure the accuracy of the information contained in this book at the time of publication.

The author disclaims any liability for any medical outcomes that may occur as a result of applying the methods suggested in this book.

Chapter 1: METALS IN THE HOME

The first step to any detoxification protocol is to reduce your overall exposure to toxic substances. To help us do that, this chapter contains examples of the heavy metals you are most likely to come into contact within your home. Some of these may surprise you, and I'm pretty sure some will shock you to the core!

At this point, it's important to note that not all heavy metals are truly toxic, while others will destroy your health faster than you can say accelerated aging and memory loss. Some of the more dangerous metals have been linked to Alzheimer's disease, epilepsy, multiple sclerosis, depression, behavioral problems, joint pain, fatigue, anxiety, kidney disease, and Parkinson's disease. The list goes on and on.

To help you understand what's happening here, it's important to note that the brain has a protective layer around it known as the blood-brain barrier. Its purpose is to keep toxins out. Unfortunately, metals such as lead, aluminum, and mercury cross that barrier with ease (we'll cover this in more detail later.) When the blood-brain barrier is breached, dangerous metals can reach parts of the brain. Over time, accumulation can lead to a range of degenerative diseases. Cognitive disorders, mental anguish, anxiety, and chronic depression may also follow.

Heavy metals such as mercury, lead, aluminum, arsenic, and cadmium like to hide in plain sight in our everyday lives. And if we aren't paying close attention, we may inadvertently *pay* to bring them into our homes! What follows is by no means a complete list, but it does serve as a valuable aid to anyone looking to reduce the number of heavy metals from his or her home. To get the ball rolling see if you can spot the heavy metal hiding in the following photo.

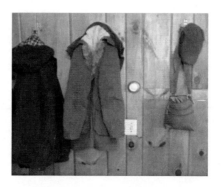

If you managed to spot this toxic invader, top marks for observation. If not, I'll give you the correct answer right before this chapter ends. For now, let's dive in by exploring some common heavy metals that most of us are exposed to. The first on our list is lead.

LEAD

Lead is a neurotoxin. A neurotoxin acts on the nervous system and disrupts the normal function of nerve cells. This makes developing fetuses and small children particularly susceptible to the dangers of lead. Lead is also associated with major depression, reduced IQ, and anxiety disorders. *Here's why…*

Lead can enter your home in various ways. One of these ways is through the waterline. If you think this only happened in Flint, Michigan, then, unfortunately, you would be wrong. Right up until 1986, lead solder was still being used to join copper pipes together. Today, plumbers use a form of lead-free solder, but many older homes still have a trace amount of lead somewhere in the waterline.

When water sits in copper pipes for any length of time, the lead used to join the pipes can break down. It then makes its way to your kitchen sink or bathtub. As we shower, heat opens up our pores, allowing trace amounts of toxins to be absorbed through the skin. There are a couple of workarounds that can help reduce the amount of lead (and other toxins) coming into your home via the waterline. First, always let the water run for a few minutes before using it. Second, add a water filter to your home. Without a water filter, your kidneys become the filter!

There are lots of water filters on the market, and some are better quality than others. As with most things, you tend to get what you pay for. If cost is a consideration, know that ***any filter is better than no filter at all.***

Two water filter companies worth checking out are Berkey water filters and Pure Effect filters. I have no affiliation with either, I'm simply trying to save you some time. A Berkey water filter is a standalone unit that usually sits on the top of the kitchen counter. Simply add suspect water to it, which then filters down and supplies fresh drinking water whenever you need it. By comparison, a Pure Effects filter attaches directly to the kitchen faucet and has an option to mount the filter on the countertop or under the sink. Installation is pretty basic, and most homeowners should be able to complete it *without* the need to hire a plumber.

If you suspect lead is somewhere along your waterline, it pays to have your water tested by a professional. Having your water tested is relatively easy and inexpensive to do. A small sample is collected from each faucet and those samples are sent away to a lab. A quick Google search will give you a list of people who perform water testing in your area.

Homes that are completely free of lead pipes aren't completely off the hook. Some towns and cities across the US often have an aging network of pipes hidden somewhere underground. If it makes you feel better, this is a problem that dates back to Roman times. As the Empire spread, so did the use of lead pipes. It's speculated that lead plumbing had an impact on the minds of Roman leaders. Alas, five hundred years later and history seems to be repeating itself!

Okay, moving along nicely, lead can also be found on the glaze of ceramic dishes. Colored dishware tends to have more glaze while white dishes contain the least. This is good to know when buying new dishware. Those that are of higher quality often contain no lead at all.

Lead can also be found in spices such as turmeric, chili powder, and paprika. Whoa! Isn't turmeric supposed to be good for you? Yes, but many spices now coming from India and China contain alarmingly high levels of lead!

Lead paint is something most of us are aware of, but it's the fine dust particles that cause the real problem. These can linger in the home long after a remodeling project is complete. When this happens, those tiny particles have a way of finding their way into our bodies, causing serious neurologic changes, developmental delays, and irritability. Lead tends to accumulate in the body (even small amounts), hence those fine dust particles pose a serious health risk to young children. High levels of lead may even be fatal! If you are attempting a small DIY project, be sure to wet the whole area down and wear a mask. If in doubt, consult an expert. For larger projects, you will need to hire a licensed contractor to do the work for you.

Lead can even show up at your front door gift-wrapped. Many imported toys have high levels of lead that you really wouldn't want young children sucking on. If you are about to send someone a birthday present, it's best to check reviews BEFORE buying. If you want a truly lead-free gift, you could always try spending the same amount of money on a memorable experience. It's funny how kids will remember a day at the park long after a plastic toy hits the trash can.

As a side note, apple pectin has an affinity for lead and may be helpful when taken in a supplement form. For those already dealing with exposure to lead, it's also important to work with an informed healthcare provider.

You can also go deeper with this topic by following "Lead Safe Mama" on her Facebook page. It's a good resource for tracking lead that can be hidden in a wide range of products.

CADMIUM

Cadmium is classified as a known human carcinogen (cancer-causing). It can also cause damage to the kidneys and lungs. Other symptoms to be aware of are nausea, vomiting, diarrhea, unhealthy weight loss, and hypertension. Cadmium can also have an impact on the skeletal system.

Exposure to cadmium mainly occurs from the consumption of contaminated foods. That said, modern manufacturing techniques ensure there is no shortage of cadmium in our lives. It's present in batteries, synthetic rubber mats, and even copy machines! At this point, I'd like to remind you that the aim of this chapter *isn't* to make you feel overwhelmed, **it's to make you aware.** Rest assured, there are lots of practical solutions coming later in the book.

Cadmium is also something to be aware of for those living near hazardous waste facilities such as junkyards, recycling centers, or places where smelting activities are carried out.

Cadmium can also be found in tobacco smoke (which obviously includes passive inhalation).

ALUMINUM

Aluminum is another neurotoxin; it can sneak past the blood-brain barrier with ease. Many studies have linked aluminum to Alzheimer's and

Parkinson's disease. Here are a few ways it can get into your system.

Cooking with aluminum pots and pans can add it to your food. Some estimates suggest upwards of 2 mg per meal. Is that enough to cause a mental decline? Who knows, but what we do know is aluminum accumulates over time. Perhaps this is why we see so much Alzheimer's later in life.

Either way, the safer option is to switch any aluminum pots and pans you may have to stainless steel ones. When roasting in the oven, try using a glass Pyrex dish or stainless-steel grilling basket. Both of these will also reduce the amount of aluminum foil you use.

Staying in the kitchen, certain foods, such as processed cheeses contain aluminum-based food additives. Some brands of baking powder also contain aluminum, while others are 100% aluminum-free. It pays to make a habit of reading food labels. This can help prevent sneaky amounts of aluminum from entering your bloodstream. If enough of us stop buying toxic products, the stores will stop selling them. Voting with your wallet lets the supermarket know which brands suck and which to keep stocked on the shelf.

Believe it or not, aluminum can also be found in toothpaste, cosmetics, and underarm antiperspirants. Aluminum salts are used to plug up pores so that you won't sweat as much. Deodorants, on the other hand, have no aluminum. They work by reducing body odor with either fragrance or antibacterial compounds. The foods we eat can also have an impact on body odor.

Soda companies use aluminum cans to package their products. They are quick to assure us that drinking out of aluminum cans is safe. And while this may (or may not) be true the best way to limit your risk is to drink less soda. Soda is a burden on the immune system which will hinder the detoxification process.

MERCURY

Mercury is yet another heavy metal that crosses the blood-brain barrier. It should come as no surprise that it's also linked to mental problems such as anxiety and depression. But there's more to this heavy metal than meets the eye. Mercury is a naturally occurring, toxic heavy metal. When it reacts with another substance, it forms a compound.

These compounds can be expressed in various ways. To keep things simple, let's look at mercury in three forms.

1. Elemental (or metallic) mercury.

2. Inorganic mercury compounds.

3. Organic mercury compounds (which form methylmercury).

ELEMENTAL MERCURY

Elemental mercury is a shiny, silver-white metal that is liquid at room temperature. Elemental mercury is an element that has not reacted with another substance. It's sometimes found in thermometers, fluorescent light bulbs, and some electrical switches.

When elemental mercury is placed inside glass, it poses little threat so long as the glass remains intact. However, if the glass is accidentally broken, elemental mercury can become an issue. Once it hits the floor, it will immediately break down into smaller droplets. These droplets can disappear through small cracks in baseboards or floorboards.

At room temperature, these droplets evaporate and become a toxic vapor. Vapors are absorbed via the respiratory tract and distributed throughout the body. Elemental mercury is also used in dental amalgams, which then becomes a part of you 24/7. When teeth are exposed to heat or chewing dental amalgams release a toxic vapor. Despite this, the ADA (American Dental Association) continues to assure people that silver/mercury fillings are safe. *Me? I'm not so sure.*

If your dentist is telling you that silver/mercury amalgams are completely safe, then perhaps it's time to look for a new dentist. If you already have dental amalgams a specialized dentist is required to remove them (more on this later).

INORGANIC MERCURY

Inorganic mercury compounds are formed when mercury combines with other elements, such as sulfur or oxygen. Inorganic mercury compounds can occur naturally in the environment in the form of mercury salts. Generally, they are white powder or crystals, except for mercuric sulfide (cinnabar) which is red. Most uses of inorganic compounds have been discontinued, although some are still used by industry to make other chemicals.

ORGANIC MERCURY

Organic mercury compounds are formed when mercury combines with carbon. This can happen during the coal burning process. Working on the principle that what goes up must come down, we can assume that once mercury is released into the air, it will eventually settle on land or sea. It then reacts with bacteria to form a toxic form of mercury known as methylmercury.

Methylmercury then works its way up the food chain to you. Fish that feed on smaller fish such as mackerel, marlin, orange roughy, shark, swordfish, tilefish, ahi tuna, and bigeye tuna all contain higher levels. Smaller fish such as anchovies and sardines tend to fare much better. Sardines are perhaps your best bet as they contain trace amounts of selenium. Selenium limits the adverse effects of methylmercury, and we'll also cover this in more detail later.

Methylmercury is the major source of organic mercury found in humans.
Methylmercury isn't something to take lightly. Poisoning from methylmercury can manifest itself in more ways than you or I can shake a stick at. As levels in the body rise, more symptoms appear. These can include devastating neurological damage, memory problems, anxiety, depression, etc.

Methylmercury is toxic to the central and peripheral nervous systems. It can also have a serious impact on the immune system, lungs, kidneys, and digestive system.

Methylmercury is the one to watch out for, as it is the most common form of organic mercury compound found in the environment. Like most heavy metals, it also accumulates in the body over time. During pregnancy, methylmercury can pass from mother to baby. It's also linked to developmental abnormalities and cerebral palsy.

Good to know: From a toxicity perspective, methylmercury (from fish consumption) and elemental mercury (found in dental amalgams) eclipse all other forms. Yes, mercury can be found in a wide range of other places (including some medical products) but your biggest danger comes from a buildup of methylmercury and elemental mercury. The good news is, the detoxification process laid out in this book can be applied to ALL forms of mercury.

ARSENIC

Arsenic is known to cause an increase in lung, bladder, and skin cancers. Arsenic is a metalloid, meaning it can exhibit some properties of metals and non-metals. It finds its way into air, food, soil, and groundwater, the latter being the most common.

As such, arsenic can be found in private well water, some seafood, rice, and rice-based food products. Rice tends to absorb more arsenic, as it tends to grow best in flooded rice fields. And while an occasional bowl of rice is unlikely to cause any lasting problems, it is something to be aware of if you consume rice regularly.

If this is you, here's the workaround.

1: Soak rice overnight,

2: Drain the rice and rinse thoroughly with fresh water. This opens up the grain and allows arsenic to be washed out. Sprouted Blonde Rice (grown locally in California) seems to fare much better.

At one time, wood preservers accounted for almost 90% of arsenic produced domestically. By 2004, many manufacturers transitioned away from arsenic trioxide. This was in response to customer demand, which just goes to show the power of voting with your wallet.

Pressure-treated decks built before this date may still contain arsenic. This is something to think about when standing barefoot on your deck. Lest we forget, arsenic is also used in weed killers and rat poison!

Okay, before we end this chapter did you manage to spot the heavy metal in the photo? Let's take a closer look at that innocent-looking thermostat on the wall.

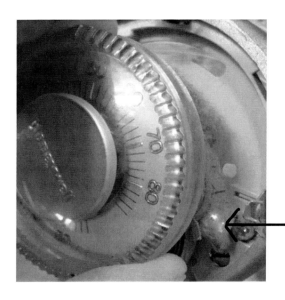

Here we see an example of elemental mercury in all its splendor! As mentioned earlier, thermostats such as these become problematic if the glass is broken. At room temperature, this could allow toxic vapors to be inhaled.

If you come across one of these in your home, it's best to seal it in a plastic container and call your local transfer station. They can usually help you dispose of it.

Bottom line: When heavy metals overwhelm the body, health problems can often intensify. Because of their high degree of toxicity, arsenic, cadmium, chromium, lead, and mercury all play a significant role in mental health.

Chapter 2: WHEN HEAVY METALS BECOME KRYPTONITE

Dealing with a heavy metals issue can be an overwhelming experience. At times, the information we need can be difficult to find and even more difficult to understand. *How do I know this?*

In 2011, I became seriously ill. By 2012, I was stuck in a wheelchair. To add to my problems, conventional medicine seemed to be making matters worse. Thankfully, I'm a persistent person, it's just in my nature. Rather than give up, I became better informed. I took my health into my own hands and today I am healthy and walking again. I take ZERO medications and my energy keeps me going until midnight. I also make a point of running up staircases. Not too shabby for a man that couldn't walk.

When you give the body what it needs, and steer it away from what it doesn't, a healing opportunity presents itself. In simple terms, the toxins must come out, and nutrients must flow in. The body will do the rest for you.

As a result of my earlier illness, I now have a much better understanding of what it is like to be trapped inside a sickly body and desperate for answers. Back then, I noticed those who understood the detox process presented it like they had swallowed a medical textbook. For the average layperson, the information might as well be written in a foreign language. Long story short, once I got back on my feet, I wanted to give something back.

I wrote this book intending to make the detoxification process easier to understand. My goal was to turn a complicated process into something interesting and relatable. In short, this book serves as a buffer between the layperson, and the information held by those who understand it.

Let's jump into our next topic, ready?

At some point, your body is going to come into direct contact with a toxic heavy metal, no question about it. How well you handle that exposure depends on the following three things.

..

1. The substance.

2. The amount of time spent coming into contact with it.

3. Your ability to detoxify it.

Trace amounts of heavy metals routinely turn up in fruit juice, medications, health supplements, and even baby formula! And yet, when we look at the Earth's crust as a whole, these heavy metals were once relatively scarce. *Ever wonder how we got here?*

The link between heavy metals and serious health problems has its roots in the industrial revolution. Back then, techniques used in manufacturing allowed metals to seep into our waterways, our soil, and the air we breathe. It's fair to assume that our ancestors might not have realized the long-term implications of dumping heavy metals into the environment. Today, such ignorance is no longer an acceptable excuse.

Yet corporations around the world continue to add toxic materials to our daily products. It's now commonplace to find lead in lipstick, cadmium in car seat covers, aluminum in food products, and the list goes on and on and on.

As a result, getting metals into the body is the easy part. And while a lot can be said for eating healthy, no amount of kale soup is going to chelate heavy metals. As mentioned in the introduction, organic food is tested for pesticides, *not* heavy metals.

Unraveling the damage caused by heavy metals now becomes a process. Not least because symptoms present themselves in multiple forms. Once we have one health-destroying heavy metal floating around inside us, the risk of accumulating another increases tenfold.

The difference between sickness and health comes down to how effective your body is at filtering out toxins. Taking the biggest hit for the team is the liver and kidneys. But there's a problem lurking, can you see it?

Earlier, we learned that the brain doesn't have a filter; it has a protective barrier around it. Heavy metals such as lead, mercury, and aluminum can sneak past that barrier with ease. Once they get inside the brain, your pituitary gland is left exposed.

THE PITUITARY GLAND

This small gland is only about the size of a pea, but it plays a pivotal role in your health. The pituitary gland is often described as the "master gland."

Why?

The hormones the pituitary gland helps to create have an impact on other parts of the endocrine system. This would include the thyroid, adrenal glands, ovaries, and testes. Before we give all the credit to the pituitary gland, it's worth mentioning that it gets a little help from the hypothalamus. The hypothalamus signals to the pituitary gland when to stimulate or inhibit hormone production. Stay with me here because the importance of knowing this is about to link right back to heavy metals.

The pituitary gland is a key player in producing melatonin. Melatonin is the hormone that regulates sleep-wake cycles. As we sleep, our bodies do a great deal of detoxifying. Without sleep, the brain cannot rest or repair itself. To be clear, sleep is an essential part of detoxification.

SLEEP

As we sleep, our brains shrink, allowing cerebrospinal fluid to flood the area and clear out harmful toxins. It's the equivalent of a cleanup crew coming to clean the store after hours. Recent research suggests people who sleep better have a reduced risk of Alzheimer's disease. The thinking behind this is that harmful waste proteins linked to Alzheimer's are washed away as we sleep.

Heavy metals such as mercury, aluminum, and lead unnaturally stimulate the pituitary. This might explain why some folks feel "tired and wired" at bedtime. It can also feel like the mind "chatter" just won't shut off.

The pituitary gland also plays a key role in our intuition. When our intuition is off, we lose the ability to sense when something is immediately and instinctively wrong.

Let's explore this a little.

When heavy metals are present in the brain, rational thinking becomes an unachievable skill. At best, foggy thinking becomes the new normal; at worst, a person is capable of lashing out in either anger or frustration. Perhaps both are consequences of a mind that is slowly being poisoned. Clearly, the human mind cannot cope with heavy metal exposure hence the importance of detoxification cannot be understated.

THE WEAKEST LINK

Unfortunately, it's not just the brain that's left exposed to toxic metals. Heavy metals can settle just about anywhere in the body. Be it in the thyroid, prostate, heart, muscle, or even bone. When heavy metals settle in their new home, they do a first-class job of messing with body chemistry.

How so?

To the body, heavy metals look similar to many important minerals. As an example, thallium mimics potassium which can affect the nerves and cardiovascular system. Cadmium is known to displace zinc, and lead is so chemically similar to calcium that it leaches into the bones. Here's the huge takeaway message. This process happens faster in a body that is deficient in minerals.

Minerals help to perform functions necessary for life. The five major minerals in the human body are calcium, phosphorus, potassium, sodium, and magnesium. These minerals were once found in abundance in the foods we ate. Unfortunately, we now live in a world where food is grown for profit, rather than mineral content.

Trace minerals that your body needs to stay healthy are becoming harder to find. This can cause a real disconnect between chronic illness (illness lasting three months or more) and missing minerals. In case you missed it, heavy metals are masters of mimicry. To simplify, they are fake minerals that confuse the body.

WHEN SILVER BECOMES MERCURY

We touched on dental amalgam earlier, let's recap, define exactly what they are, and why they present a problem. Dental amalgam (also known as silver fillings) is a material used to fill cavities. It's a mixture of metals consisting of silver, tin, copper, and elemental mercury. The latter making up as much as 50% of the filling.

Once the amalgam becomes an integral part of the tooth, mercury vapors begin to trickle down into the rest of the body. This happens around the clock,

365 days a year. Over time, this build up causes a cascade of health problems. The only way to prevent further exposure is to remove the "silver" fillings. But as always, the devil is in the details.

Before attempting to remove a silver filling, it's important to find an educated dentist who fully understands the dangers of mercury toxicity. Sadly, most do not. In the *wrong* hands, removal will often create more problems than it solves.

Heavy metals experts around the world agree that these types of fillings should have been banned years ago. Despite a mountain of evidence alerting dentists to the dangers, some continue putting "silver" fillings into the mouths of children. The argument often put forward is that metal fillings are stronger and last longer. *Sheesh, thanks for nothing!*

But as we learned earlier, mercury isn't confined to teeth. It should come as no surprise that some of the highest readings are found in our waterways. As such, the higher up the food chain you go the higher the concentration of methylmercury. Consumable products made from fish can also become a problem. Inexpensive fish oil supplements sold in some big box stores can be a hidden source of methylmercury. Some of the more reputable supplement companies offer third-party testing. Third-party testing ensures that someone who is perceived to be independent checks the fish for excessive levels of methylmercury.

FURTHER DISRUPTION

Remember, what heavy metals do best is cause disruption. It's their party piece, if you like. We've already learned that they like to mimic important minerals and just for good measure, heavy metals also mess up enzyme activity.

Enzymes help regulate different processes in the body. They also make certain chemical reactions happen. Whenever a cell needs something done in a hurry, it uses enzymes to speed up chemical reactions. Enzymes are special types of proteins. Like all proteins, they are made from strings of amino acids. Inside the amino acid, cysteine group is the sulfhydryl group.

Why is this important to know?

Sulfhydryl groups are good at moving electrons around and holding the good metals like copper and zinc in place. Unfortunately, old friend mercury also likes to link up with sulfhydryl groups. Once mercury gets attached, it displaces the copper or the zinc that was supposed to be there.

ZINC AND COPPER

Zinc is important as it's required for the catalytic activity of more than three-hundred enzymes. It's also involved in the synthesis and metabolism of carbohydrates, fats, proteins, nucleic acids, and other micronutrients. Zinc is an immune-system booster that helps the body stay healthy. But everything it's a delicate balancing act. Copper and zinc have an interesting relationship. The intake of one causes the other to decrease in the body. A healthy balance between the two is critically important to prevent a buildup of toxicity in the body. Copper is important for a healthy heart, bones, and brain development. Copper and zinc are a team that likes to work together. But those destructive heavy metals we keep talking about cause this fine balance to become unglued.

Are we there yet?

Yes, copper and zinc are important, but so are all the other minerals. As an example, the heart needs calcium, magnesium, and potassium or it simply won't pump smoothly. Let's not forget, heart disease is the number one killer in the US. When heavy metals mimic essential minerals, they prevent them from doing their job. When this happens, **heavy metals will send every system in the body out of balance.**

BRAIN FOG AND FATIGUE

Now, can you imagine the complexity of the problem once heavy metals cross the blood-brain barrier and enter the mind? Can we expect to see a little brain fog? *I think so.*

I'm sure many have heard the term "mad as a hatter". A reference to English hat makers who, not so long ago, used mercury as part of their hat-making process. These craftsmen were well known for their irrational outbursts and depressive bouts. Once mercury entered the bloodstream, it was only a matter of time before it crossed the blood-brain barrier.

Alas, problems aren't limited to mental anguish or brain fog. Once heavy metals disrupt enzyme production, essential nutrients are blocked from reaching the mitochondria (we'll cover these little powerhouses in more detail later). Think of them as the battery inside your watch. When the battery runs down the watch slowly runs down. When the mitochondria are disrupted, people will often complain of debilitating fatigue.

By now you should be realizing that heavy metals do a pretty good job of messing with all aspects of our health. But without a clear plan, heavy metals can be an extremely complicated riddle to solve. With that in mind, the next chapter will show you how to test yourself for heavy metals.

Chapter 3: TESTING FOR HEAVY METALS

As with any test, it pays to be your own advocate. If you go into this blind, then you are simply hoping that the person doing the testing knows what they are doing. Rest assured, by the time you have finished this short chapter you will have a clear understanding of what each test involves.

Okay, if you have been paying close attention, you may have noticed that heavy metals are an insidious, omnipresent part of everyday life. They are inside our homes and they are inside us. So, if we already know this, then you might be asking what's the point of testing? That's a great question, and I like the way you think. *Here's the short answer …*

When the body is unable to filter out toxins, it stores them away for another time. This build-up is reflected in our hair, blood, and stool. A sample allows us to see just how well your body is (or isn't) detoxifying itself.

Knowing just how many heavy metals are in our bodies can be quite revealing. Having this information moving forward also makes treatment protocols more effective. For anyone with an ongoing health issue (but without a firm diagnosis), this could be your lightbulb moment!

There are several test options available. The most common being hair, blood and urine. Each offers a snapshot in time. Hair tends to reflect a period of months. Blood and urine tend to be weeks and hours, respectively.

The most accurate result comes from combining tests, which are sometimes known as "tri-testing." In this chapter, we'll walk you through the pros and cons of each. But first, it's important to note that toxicity, mineral depletion, and sickness all go hand in hand.

If we know that to be true, we would expect to see higher levels of heavy metals in our test results, **but that's not always the case.** There are other factors to take into consideration. For example, when the body becomes too ill or too weak to detoxify it can hold on to metals by storing them in fat tissue. This is important information to have under your belt, as the person reading your results may jump to the wrong conclusions. Looking at the data, subjectively leads us to first ask—is this person's detoxification pathway overtaxed?

Don't panic if you aren't sure what detoxification pathways are, there's a whole chapter dedicated to the subject later in the book. For now, let's not go off on too many tangents because I'd like for us to stay focused on testing. Without further ado, let's dive into the world of heavy metals testing!

THE HAIR ANALYSIS TEST

The hair analysis test is noninvasive and relatively inexpensive. At the time of writing, it can be purchased for around $125. Some states may require a physician to order the test for you, others do not, and you can simply order the test online.

As the name suggests, a hair analysis test requires a hair sample. This is usually done from home and full instructions come with the kit. Once a hair sample is collected, it is then sent to a lab in a prepaid envelope.

The hair analysis test can detect a wide range of metals such as lead, cadmium, arsenic, and mercury. It's very effective at picking up on mercury found in fish, but not so accurate at showing dental mercury. For this reason, it can be helpful to have someone interpret the test results for you. Overall, the hair analysis test is a great go-to test, but it's by no means a definitive test.

The hair analysis test can also provide valuable data regarding your trace mineral levels. Without wanting to sound like a broken record, minerals are important for maintaining health. Without sufficient minerals, the body's detoxification process will run below par. As a side note, when minerals are in short supply, vitamins are poorly absorbed.

CHALLENGE TEST (URINE)

A challenge test is sometimes touted as the gold standard by the medical profession, but that's not to say it's problem-free. In fact, in the wrong hands, it can do a great deal of harm. *Here's why...*

The challenge test is looking for heavy metals that pass in the urine. Prior to the test, a baseline sample is taken.

Next, a pharmaceutical-grade chelator is given (such as EDTA, DMSA, or DMPS). A chelator, sometimes called a chelating agent, is any substance whose molecules can form several bonds to a single metal ion. In plain English, a chelating agent sticks to certain heavy metals in the hope of flushing them out as you pee.

Once the chelating agent flushes out heavy metals, the pee is again collected and measured. These results are then compared to the previous baseline numbers. *So far, so good, but there is a problem. Can you see it?*

If a patient's kidneys *aren't* functioning optimally, a challenge test may produce a false-negative. Put simply, heavy metals are moving around the body, but not necessarily out of the body. This can also leave a patient feeling pretty crappy after the test.

The added downside of this test is anyone with impaired kidney function will not be able to fully excrete metals. In this case, a significant risk of kidney damage should be taken into account (particularly in older individuals). If the situation allows, it's always prudent to allow an unwell patient to stabilize before making ANY attempts to flush out heavy metals. Sadly, there are some in the medical field who seem to overlook this simple principle. Or as my old mom used to say, "common sense isn't that common."

BLOOD TEST

Depending on the type of exposure, heavy metals can remain at high levels in the blood for about a week. After that, they tend to gravitate to other areas of the body. Standard testing for mercury looks at the total amount of mercury in the blood. The problem with this can be twofold. First, the type of mercury found in fish will almost certainly dominate the test, causing a series of skewed results. Second, when results are overwhelmed by fish mercury, it's difficult to estimate how much mercury is leaching into the body from dental fillings.

Here's the workaround: Separating blood samples into two separate reference ranges gives a much clearer picture. This allows us to see how much mercury is being accumulated from each form of mercury, be it fish mercury (AKA methylmercury) or dental mercury (AKA elemental mercury).

THE IMPORTANCE OF TRI-TESTING.

Dental mercury is predominantly excreted through the kidneys. When the two blood samples are cross-referenced with urine results, it can show just how well (or poorly) the kidneys are working. And when blood samples from fish-based mercury are compared to a hair sample, it reveals how well the person is detoxifying fish mercury.

To simplify, the blood can capture both forms of mercury (be it from fish or dental). When each blood sample is cross-referenced with urine tests, it's an indication of how much dental mercury is being excreted. When the blood tests are cross-referenced with the hair sample, it shows how well fish mercury is being excreted. *Now, can you see why tri-testing is so important?*

With these pieces of the puzzle in place, a detoxification program can now be tailored to suit your individual needs.

Those who aren't mobilizing metals optimally via the liver and kidneys are the ones who will be the most difficult to treat. In this case, readings of metals may be lower as the body attempts to hold on to them by sending them into fat storage.

It's worth mentioning that some metals are excreted in the stool, but again, this is limited to the person's ability to detoxify. In this case, supporting the detoxification pathways becomes key (more on this in the coming chapter).

DON'T BE GREEDY

As we move through this book, I'd like you to be thinking about the golden rule of detoxification, which is this: Whenever an attempt is made to remove toxins from the body, don't be greedy. This simply means that chelation (removal of metals) has to be done slowly. Detoxification isn't a sprint, it's a marathon race. Any attempt to do this too quickly will cause you to crash and burn. Trust me, I've been there, and you don't want that.

Chapter 4: DETOXIFICATION PATHWAYS

In its most basic form, detoxification is the process of removing harmful substances from the body. Toxins come out via six main pathways, but over time, these pathways may become sluggish and less efficient. Fatigue sets in and brain fog becomes the new normal.

Here comes some good news!

When the body's detoxification pathways are working optimally, thinking becomes clearer, energy skyrockets, and a peaceful night's sleep becomes achievable. *No, really, it's true.*

Sleep is a pretty big deal as the body detoxifies best when it's in rest and digest mode. We'll cover sleep in more detail in the following chapter. For now, I'd like to show you what these six pathways are, what can go wrong with them, and more importantly, how to keep them running smoothly! Doing most of the heavy lifting is the liver. But the kidneys, skin, lungs, lymphatic system, and the digestive system all play an important role too. Let's kick off with the lungs because it only takes a few seconds to realize what a pivotal role they play in keeping us alive.

LUNGS

As you read this, take a deep breath. Now hold it until you finish the next three paragraphs. *By my count, it's less than thirty seconds, ready?*

Generally speaking, the lungs do an exceptional job of keeping harmful contaminants at bay. Problems arise when exposure to a harmful substance is either prolonged or poisonous. Cadmium and arsenic are two such substances. Both of these can be found in cigarette smoke.

Damage to the lungs runs by the name of pulmonary toxicity, or lung toxicity. Toxic mold spores, ammonia, and asbestos will all do the trick too. Signs that something untoward is happening in the lungs can be shortness of breath and coughing. Anything that lasts more than a few days is worth getting checked out by your medical provider. Mold can be a little trickier, as many doctors won't pick up on the connection. There's also no blood test for mold toxicity, which makes it a hidden, stealthy type of infection.

Make no mistake, mold is the ugly sister to heavy metals. Both can shut down your detoxification pathways and in doing so, will mimic symptoms of anxiety, fatigue, and brain fog. You can find helpful solutions to mold in my book titled "Toxic Mold Book."

We sometimes think of the lungs as two bags of air. This couldn't be further from the truth. A much better mental image would be to think of them as a highly sophisticated pair of sponges, each being gently squeezed. Oxygen is fed to the lungs via a series of tubes that become increasingly smaller. These tubes look a lot like roots you might find under a large tree, getting gradually smaller the deeper they go.

If you made it to this point without gasping for air, congrats! Hopefully, this short exercise made you realize just how important your lungs are.

HELP FOR POORLY FUNCTIONING LUNGS

Illness aside, making life easier for the lungs is relatively easy and inexpensive to do. The fastest way to do this is to clean up your indoor air quality. This can be done by simply adding plants to your home.

NASA has undertaken quite a bit of research in this area and found that Peace Lily, Mother-in-Law's Tongue, and Ivy were all ideal candidates for this purpose. Compared to other indoor plants these are also pretty low maintenance making them a WIN/WIN.

Air fresheners, on the other hand, are notorious for irritating the delicate lining of the lungs (as are most household sprays). Indoor air quality can be greatly improved by simply opening windows whenever possible.

If your situation allows, spend less time sitting indoors and more time outside in the fresh air. To help alleviate any minor respiratory conditions, Mullein tea can also be helpful as it helps to lubricate the delicate lining of the lung.

If you have pine trees, growing locally, be sure to walk among them breathing in that rich pine scent. As you do, your airways will automatically open up and the air quality will feel better. The healing benefit of pine is well documented and dates back to ancient times. If pine trees aren't an option, then the next best thing is to use a quality pine-tree essential oil. Adding a few drops to a diffuser can help to bring relief. That said, steer well clear of bargain-priced oils or even worse fake pine in the form of scented air fresheners. They are toxic to your body.

SKIN

Your skin is alive and intelligent. It doesn't take kindly to being clogged up with makeup, perfumes, or even worse bug-spray! Lest we forget, the skin is porous. **Whatever goes onto the skin goes into the skin,** which then travels into the bloodstream. Problems begin when the number of toxins being absorbed into the skin becomes greater than the body's ability to detoxify them. Be aware of this when using budget soaps and shampoos in the shower. Heat opens up the pores, making it easier for toxins to pass through the skin.

On a hot summer day, be aware that the skin needs to breathe. Wrapping it in layers of nylon fibers only makes this more difficult. Wearing natural fibers such as cotton and hemp, allows the skin to breathe. Keeping yourself properly hydrated is critically important especially in the heat of the day.

Skin is sometimes described as the third kidney. It's also the body's largest organ. Psoriasis, eczema, and rashes are all indicators that your skin is struggling to cope with something inside the body. Adding cream to the area may help short term, but it *doesn't* address the root cause.

HELP FOR YOUR SKIN

Toxins can be drawn out of the skin by applying a thin layer of natural clay. Bentonite clay can be purchased online or through your local health food store. Preparation is super easy to do, simply mix it with water to make a paste. For a facemask, apply it to the face and leave it to dry for about fifteen minutes. Other areas can be left on a little longer, so long as it doesn't feel uncomfortable. Once you are finished, wash the clay off with warm water.

Brushing the skin daily with a firm, natural bristle brush will boost circulation. This, in turn, stimulates the lymphatic system (more on this in a moment). The ideal time to brush the skin is first thing in the morning (before you shower). Start with the feet and work your way up to your legs, then hands and arms working towards the heart.

In the evening, adding a cup of Epsom salts along with one cup of organic apple cider vinegar to hot bath water will draw toxins out of the skin. By far the most effective way to help your skin release toxins is to use a sauna. Bonus points if it's a far infrared sauna that will speed up the elimination of heavy metals. Rather than overwhelm you, we'll touch on saunas again later in the book.

KIDNEYS

The primary role of the kidneys is to filter blood. Kidneys can filter as much as 150 liters of blood per day! Anything deemed suspect is removed from the blood and sent out to the bladder. But that's not all kidneys do. They also balance blood pressure, maintain proper electrolyte levels, and balance the pH of the blood to name but a few functions.

We each have two kidneys which are made up of about a million nephrons. Nephrons are a network of tiny tubes that make for a pretty delicate filtering system. Under normal circumstances, these remarkable filters give us good service day in day out. However, some substances can be poisonous to the kidneys. Chemical solvents, heavy metals, and certain medications are all especially harmful to the kidneys.

The term "nephrotoxicity," simply means toxicity in the kidneys. Kidneys can handle a certain amount of nephrotoxins, but *continued* exposure will result in damage. In some circumstances, this damage can be irreversible or even deadly!

Other causes of kidney damage can be linked to diabetes and poorly managed high blood pressure. Early signs that something untoward is happening in the kidneys are an increase in urination. Urine may also appear foamy or bubbly due to a higher than normal amount of protein being excreted.

Puffiness under the eyes, sudden fatigue, excessive foot odor, and/or swelling in the ankles can all be indicators that something isn't quite right in the kidney department. If you suspect you have any type of kidney issue be sure to get it checked out by your healthcare provider.

HELP FOR YOUR KIDNEYS

Hydration is key to kidney health. Adding freshly squeezed lemon juice to a morning glass of water can help with this. For best results, always drink lemon water at room temperature on an empty stomach. Bonus points if you have access to clean spring water. If not, try cutting out the plastic bottle by filtering your own water – water filters were covered earlier in the book.

Diuretics can help increase the amount of urine that your kidneys produce. This can be helpful when trying to flush the urinary system (more on this later). Diuretics do this by altering the body's electrolyte or body salt compositions. Obviously, it's important to be drinking enough water to help keep you hydrated. There are lots of diuretics out there, but I like natural ones such as dandelion tea.

Herbs that can help cleanse the kidneys are juniper berries and uva ursi. Tea made from a large handful of dried corn silk may also prove helpful to soothe the urinary tract. That said, it pays not to overload the kidneys with too many things at once. As with anything new, better to start with a small dose and go slow. Adding fresh parsley to your diet (or daily smoothie) can be helpful too.

The kindest thing you can do for your kidneys is to eliminate any further exposure to nephrotoxins. If your kidneys are overworked or sluggish, you may find "Rentone" (sold by Ayush Herbs) is particularly helpful.

THE LYMPHATIC SYSTEM

The lymphatic system is part of the vascular system and an important part of the immune system. It uses a fluid by the name of lymph to send infection-fighting white blood cells throughout the body. It also maintains fluid balance and plays a role in absorbing fats and fat-soluble nutrients.

There are approximately 600 checkpoints (known as lymph nodes) located at certain points around the body. The primary role of these is to check the quality of the lymph. You may have noticed how lymph nodes sometimes swell up in response to an infection. If the swelling persists, it can be cause for concern, especially when accompanied by fever or unexplained weight-loss.

When the lymphatic system becomes overburdened with too many toxins it becomes sluggish. This is sometimes described as lymphatic dysfunction. The good news is; sluggish lymph can be improved with movement (AKA exercise)

HELP FOR YOUR LYMPHATIC SYSTEM

Lymph moves best when you move. The human body was never intended to sit still for hours at a time staring at a computer screen, which is why the lymphatic system doesn't have its own pump. A brisk morning walk is enough to get things moving. Or as Hippocrates once said, "Walking is man's best medicine."

If walking isn't your thing, you can also get the lymph moving by jumping on a small rebounding trampoline. You can pick these up for under $100 and if money is tight, you can sometimes find a used one for $10 or less. Rebounding trampolines are a great way to exercise as they require no gym membership. You can even do it indoors while listening to music.

If a little light jumping while listening to music isn't your thing either, then allow me to introduce the James Bond shower.

To do this simply hop in a hot shower. Feels good, right? Okay, just before you get out, be sure to turn the water to cold. I know right, but trust me, this is one of the most effective ways to get sluggish lymph moving again.

You can start with just a few seconds and then try to work your way up to a whole minute. The more times you do this the easier it gets. A friend once asked me if doing a James Bond shower every morning would help him live longer. Without missing a beat, I said, "I can't guarantee it, but it might feel like it". Joking aside, a few seconds of cold water not only gets the lymph moving it can REALLY help to lift your mood. I guess you'll never know until you try it.

THE DIGESTIVE SYSTEM

Digestion begins with the mouth and ends with the anus. The primary role of the digestive system is to absorb nutrients and eliminate waste. When the body has everything it needs, heavy metals form part of that waste. In case you were wondering, then yes, I'm saying heavy metals leave in your poop.

The digestive system is the only system that YOU get to decide how well it works. What we put into our mouths every day is a choice. Some of those choices are nutrient dense, others, not so much.

Digestion is how the body gets those all-important minerals we mentioned earlier. Minerals are essential to help us make new cells and carry out repairs. When the body is low on minerals, it is forced to use whatever is available. Imagine trying to build a house with substandard materials. Heavy metals take this concept to a whole other level as they fool the body into thinking they are a mineral. Lead is one example of this, which is why it becomes embedded in bone.

Your digestive system is also pretty important as it's home to a whopping 70% of the immune system. Hence, it's often called "the cornerstone of good health".

HELP FOR YOUR DIGESTIVE SYSTEM

Fiber is the key to good digestion, but not everybody can tolerate fiber in the form of whole grains. Thankfully, there's no shortage of fruits and vegetables that contain fiber.

Chia seeds contain a huge amount of fiber, but they need to be soaked overnight. Soaking chia seeds in almond milk and then adding a spoonful of raw cacao powder makes chocolate chia pudding. Apples, Asian pears, and berries all have lots of fiber. And as anyone following a low-carb diet will already know, Avocado's will also do the trick.

When too many toxins find their way into the digestive tract, they are sometimes reabsorbed back into the bloodstream. Fortunately, this book will show you how excess toxins can be bound up and shipped out of the body with the use of a simple "binder".

Binders can be defined as solid, insoluble particles that pass through the gut unabsorbed. Binders attach to toxic metals and hold on to them just long enough for them to reach the toilet bowl. Chlorella, Modified Citrus Pectin, activated charcoal, Bentonite clay, Silica, and Zeolites are all binders. We'll be covering each of these in a separate chapter. Moving along nicely, let's now take a closer look at the liver.

THE LIVER

The liver is responsible for more than 500 different tasks in the body every second of every day. When it comes to multitasking, this bad boy is in a league of its own. But when it gets clogged or damaged, detoxification's efforts come to a grinding halt. The good news is the liver can literally regrow itself. *No really, it's true!*

No other body part can do this. If that didn't blow your mind imagine a surgeon looking at your left leg and saying he/she has some good news and some bad news.

The bad news is your leg needs to be cut off. But the good news is it will soon grow back. Freaky, right?

But what's really impressive is the liver remains functional while it's regrowing itself!

Here are just a few of the things your liver does …

The liver helps to filter out toxins from the body, it also plays a role in fat and carbohydrate metabolism. It does this by creating a substance known as bile, which is then stored in the gallbladder. In simple terms, bile helps to break down fat making it easier to digest.

A healthy liver can have a positive impact on the thyroid, skin, and even the immune system. The liver contains high numbers of immune cells (called Kupffer cells) which destroy any pathogens that may enter the liver from the gut.

IT'S ALSO A GIVER

When the body has sufficient vitamins, the liver will hold back vitamins A, D, E, K, and B12 for a rainy day. Yup, your liver is a giver. But it should come as no surprise that when the liver isn't happy, ain't nobody happy.

Liver problems can display themselves as irritable moods (in the old days this was often described as being "liverish"). Rage and anger are also something to be on the lookout for. Traditional Chinese Medicine describes anger as an emotion of the liver.

Other symptoms may include digestive upset, which may leave you feeling bloated to feeling sluggish after food. An increase in food intolerances, or full-blown allergies. Fatigue, headaches, low energy, difficulty getting out of bed in the morning. Constipation and diarrhea are common too (especially after eating fatty foods). Skin problems such as acne, eczema, psoriasis, etc.

When the liver is struggling to keep up with the demands being placed on it, people may have trouble sleeping, especially from midnight to 3 am. If this is you, the bitter herbs like milk thistle help to cleanse the liver.

One of the more noticeable signs of a liver problem is a yellowing of the whites of the eyes known as jaundice. Symptoms of jaundice may also include a yellow tinge to the skin, dark urine, and itchiness. An inflamed liver or obstructed bile duct can also lead to this condition.

WAYS TO HELP YOUR LIVER

In case you missed it, the liver has enough things to do. A sure way to help the liver is to lessen the burden of known stressors. The most obvious would be alcohol. When the liver tries to break down alcohol, it causes damage to its cells. As the liver quickly scrambles to repair itself, damage can be caused by inflammation and scarring

Medications can also tax the liver, so it's ALWAYS a good idea to read the insert. If you notice any of the telltale signs from above, then talk to your doctor, a substitute medication may be available. Failing that, a natural alternative may prove helpful. That said, try to steer away from some of the cheaper natural supplements on the market as many are mixed with fillers. Some of these fillers can be difficult for the liver to process.

Last but not least, it should be no surprise that processed foods can also cause problems for an overworked liver. Throw into the mix fried foods, and the health of our liver is slowly edging towards the edge of a cliff. Be especially wary of any foods cooked in oils made from corn, canola, soy, safflower, and sunflower. Healthier alternatives are coconut oil, avocado oils, butter, or ghee.

Bottom line: Treat your liver well and it will keep you well. Even if your liver has had a hard life, don't despair, the liver has the potential to regenerate itself. The trick is to give it what it needs and steer it away from what it doesn't.

Chapter 5: THE MISSING LINK - SLEEP

If you spend enough time researching heavy metals, it doesn't take long before you find yourself being taken down lots of complicated rabbit holes. In the process, the basic components of detoxification become overlooked. This is unfortunate because the person dealing with toxicity needs simple solutions rather than complicated theories. One of the most overlooked solutions is sleep. Without it, there is no detoxification.

Straight out of the gate, it's important to note that the quality of sleep is *more* important than the quantity. Depending on our age, some of us need less sleep, while others crave more. Ever wonder why teenagers are such sleepy heads?

Teenage years are such a critical time for brain development; hence they need more sleep. If you are a teenager, feel free to show this book to your mom; if you are a mom, let your teenager know that playing grand theft auto in the middle of the night isn't helping the cause. Perhaps a healthy trade-off could be an early night off the computer for a few hours of extra sleep in the morning… *just saying.'*

Either way, it's no secret that a lack of sleep makes us feel grouchy and run down. Once that happens, our problem-solving skills decrease, reasoning becomes impaired, and attention to detail is lost. On the flip side, the better we sleep the better we feel.

Your body has been using sleep to recharge, repair, and detoxify itself since the day you were born. And yet, so many of us fight the idea of going to bed at a reasonable time. So, this chapter aims to first help you appreciate the value of your sleep, and then show you ways to improve it.

Let's take a peek under the hood.

Straight out of the gate you should know that your brain is a big fat energy hog. It gobbles up a whopping 20% of your daily energy intake (even though it only makes up a teeny-weeny 2% of your body's weight).

At night, as your brain sleeps something quite remarkable happens. A cleanup crew moves in and begins washing the brain's cerebrospinal fluid. Cerebrospinal fluid is a clear liquid surrounding the brain and spinal cord. It sweeps through the brain along a series of channels that surround blood vessels. This process is managed by the brain's glial cells. Hence, science has recently defined this as the "glymphatic system."

Cleaning the brain with cerebrospinal fluid helps to remove a toxic protein called beta-amyloid from brain tissue. This bit is kind of important. Beta-amyloid is known to accumulate in the brains of patients with Alzheimer's disease!

TICK-TOCK

So, our quest for a better night's sleep begins with going to bed at a reasonable time. It's a radical step I know, especially when we are competing with that new Netflix series. I hate to point out the obvious, but if you don't take care of your body, then where are you going to live?

Let's try looking at it this way…

We all grasp the importance of recharging our cell phones at night, am I right? Then why, in this digital age, are we so quick to disregard the value of recharging our own body? Look, I get it. We can all slip into the trap of checking our email every hour on the hour. But just imagine if you saw your next-door neighbor walking outside to check his mailbox every hour. *I know right, that guy next-door is nuts!*

Since the beginning of time, the hormone melatonin has been regulating our sleep-wake cycles. This is how we evolved. Then along came the electric light bulb and things kinda got screwed up.

Here's why ...

As it gets dark outside, our brain naturally begins to produce melatonin. And when the eye senses daylight it switches off melatonin production again. That's a pretty neat trick, especially if you happen to be going through a period of evolution and you need to be alert early in the morning to hunt for food.

Can you see where I am heading with this?

Whether you like it or not, your body is programmed to go to sleep when it gets dark outside and wake up to a blue sky. It doesn't take a huge stretch of the imagination to see that the electric light bulbs mimic daylight. More so if the bulb has a blue hint to it which the brain has always associated with the morning blue sky.

It's the blue light that throws our sleep cycle into chaos. If you want to become a champion sleeper, challenge yourself to become a total blue light Nazi.

Tip - You can limit the amount of blue light that's being emitted from your computer screen by installing a free app called F.lux. This tracks the time of day in your time zone. As evening comes around, it gradually reduces the amount of blue light on your computer screen. It may seem a little odd at first, but it can serve as a helpful reminder that you should be winding down. If you decide you don't like it, you can simply uninstall it.

Street lighting streaming in through a bedroom window is something else to think about. For better sleep, blackout curtains are an inexpensive fix. If you find yourself waking in the middle of the night, don't sabotage your nighttime sleep by putting a harsh bathroom light on. Rather than disrupt melatonin, try using a small plug-in night light instead.

If the goal is to improve the quality of sleep, then let's keep this simple.

Step one is going to bed at a reasonable time.

Step two is switching off all those blue light-emitting TV and computer screens at least two hours before going to bed.

If you have been dealing with sleeping problems for any length of time, try to be aware of the things that might spook your system. For sensitive people, caffeine and certain medications can throw your sleep out.

If you find yourself waking up in the middle of the night for a snack attack, it could be a sign that your blood sugar isn't being regulated properly. If this is you, it may be helpful to eat a bowl of rice an hour before bedtime.

I'm not a fan of sleeping pills as they can leave a person feeling groggy the following day. Even worse, drug dependence can become an issue down the road. If you need a little extra help to fall asleep, try the following.

MAGNESIUM

Sustained levels of stress will deplete magnesium levels faster than a speeding ticket. If our goal is to experience better sleep, then magnesium is your friend.

Before you head off to the pharmacy to buy a box of big bulky magnesium pills, know that it isn't absorbed very well through the digestive system. The better way to get magnesium into the system is through transdermal means, this simply refers to it being absorbed through the skin.

SALT AND SODA BATHS

One way to increase your magnesium levels is to try a "salt and soda bath." To do this, simply pour a cup of quality Epsom salts into a hot bath one hour before bedtime. Add an equal amount of Arm & Hammer baking soda to the water, which also helps to drain the lymphatic system and balance your pH.

The heat from the bath allows the Epsom salts to be absorbed through the skin thus flooding the system with magnesium sulfate. Some reports suggest that a Salt and Soda bath may even be helpful to decrease radiation levels from x-rays—but that's a whole other story.

SPIKE LAVENDER

Without wanting to sound like a hippy, you could also add a few drops of lavender oil directly to your pillow. This will further aid relaxation and help reduce any nighttime anxiety. This can be particularly helpful for young children. If you want to upgrade this technique, try adding a few drops of lavender into an oil diffuser. But as always, the devil is in the details …

There are over forty-five different species of lavender with over 450 varieties, some of which can stimulate the brain! Using the wrong lavender is a common mistake that many people are unaware of. Fortunately, you don't have to be one of them. The lavender that aids sleep is called "Spike Lavender." It can also help with concentration and headaches.

CBD OIL

If you are still struggling to sleep, then it's time to bring out the big guns. CBD oil has recently become more mainstream thanks to new numerous studies linking it to a wide range of health benefits. By simply adding a few drops to the tongue, CBD oil can help ease you into a deeper sleep. Among many other benefits. CBD oil also helps to reduce stress and promotes relaxation and can help with mood stabilization.

To be clear, you cannot get high from CBD oil. (Sorry if that disappoints some readers). CBD oil is a legal derivative of cannabis; however, CBD oil can ONLY be sold with the TCH component extracted. It's the TCH is the part of cannabis that's sought after by people who are looking for a high. No TCH, no high.

If you have been dealing with sleep issues for any length of time, CBD oil can be a godsend. But as always, the devil is in the details. It all boils down to the way the oil is processed. Ideally, a non-GMO, certified organic, broad-spectrum hemp oil is the way to go. If you are just starting out, trying to find the right CBD oil can be confusing. To add to the problem, there's been a recent rush of new vendors coming to market, some good, some not so good. Rest assured, I've got you covered.

If you are looking for a CBD oil that ticks all the right boxes, then check out this link. https://detox101.thegoodinside.com/shop/product/calm-hemp-oil-750mg-full-spectrum-cbd/

It's one of the better CBD oils out there. Imagine your body waking up in the morning after a good night's sleep. CBD is a great way to restore the balance between mind and body.

BETA-1, 3D GLUCAN

If CBD oil still sounds a little too rock-and-roll for you, then we could try something that has more than fifty years of research behind it. Beta-Glucans are arguably one of the most studied naturally derived supplements on the planet.

Beta-Glucans also work as immunomodulators. This simply means they help to restore balance to the immune system. As with any product, you tend to get what you pay for. If the price is an issue, don't be afraid to try some of the less expensive brands and work your way up. When you get to a brand made by Transfer-Point, you can stop. This is one of the better Beta-Glucans.

Herbal teas can also help with sleep issues. My personal favorite is chamomile tea. Allowing the tea to steep will increase its potency. That said, it's important not to try too many things at the same time. Although a little tweaking from time to time may bring good results. *Just to be clear, I said tweaking not twerking.*

Earlier, we mentioned that the brain uses lots of energy. It gets this energy by tapping into glycogen, which is a form of sugar stored in the liver. If you find yourself constantly waking every night, try taking half a teaspoon of raw honey just before bedtime. This helps to deliver just enough energy to the brain as you sleep. For best results, be sure to use locally sourced honey.

You now have plenty of sleep tools at your disposal and I see no point in overwhelming you with more. Before we head off to our next topic, I just want to mention that long term sleep deprivation is associated with heart disease, heart attack, high blood pressure, irregular heartbeat/arrhythmias, and increased risk of stroke, diabetes, obesity, and weight gain.

Chapter 6: PRE-TOX BEFORE YOU DETOX

Now that we have our sleep under control, let's jump straight into a detox protocol, right? *Meh, not so fast Tonto.* Remember the golden rule from earlier? Yup, the one that said **detoxification is a marathon race, not a sprint.** *Here's why ...*

Over time, heavy metals can accumulate in our bodies. Sometimes this happens quickly, and sometimes it happens like a drip, drip, drip from a leaking faucet. The more toxins you have the slower you'll want to go. When the body can no longer cope, excess toxins are stored away in fat cells, muscle, and even bone. Once we open the detox floodgates, all that junk from your trunk will make a sudden dash for the exit (trust me, you don't want that).

Before we get too far into this chapter, it's worth noting that we all accumulate, store, and detoxify toxins at different rates. Slower detoxifiers usually harbor more toxins. Fortunately, these folks are pretty easy to spot.

They are the ones who have tried "everything", but nothing seems to work for them. They will often complain of stubborn weight gain (that no amount of calorie restriction will move). Taking handfuls of natural supplements only seems to make matters worse. Inevitably, they feel grumpy, irritated, and are quick to anger. These are my detox homies, yet they trust nothing and no one.

If this is you, don't lose heart. When the burden of toxicity is lifted from weary shoulders, a healthier version comes to the surface. Once the toxic metals come out, so does the sun, the sky turns blue, and people become productive, patient, fun-loving creatures once again. *No really, it's true!*

The underlying problem begins when detoxification pathways become overloaded, causing a liver misfire. This is the point where new sensitivities to chemicals, foods, mold, and natural supplements begin to surface. Mold is a pretty big deal as the detoxification pathways that transport mold, also transport heavy metals.

BLOCKED PATHWAY TEST

If you aren't sure how well your detoxification pathways are working, try this simple test.

Eat a handful of fresh cilantro and see how it makes you feel. If you notice that it gives you a headache, you feel irritated, or you have a sudden urge to punch someone in the throat, then it's safe to assume that your detox pathways aren't working optimally.

Here's what just happened.

Imagine a bucket of clean water. Then add a handful of dirt to the water and wait for it to settle at the bottom. Next, take a large wooden spoon and stir the water until it becomes cloudy. *Got the picture?*

The water represents your bloodstream, the dirt is the heavy metals stored away in your fat cells, and the spoon? Well, that's cilantro. Cilantro does a great job of stirring up heavy metals in the body. In case you missed it, cilantro *isn't* the problem, it's your current inability to detoxify heavy metals that's the problem. When detoxification pathways are working optimally, heavy metals exit the body as they should.

I know what you are thinking because I've had the same thought. Would a "binder" have helped mop up all those cilantro induced heavy metals? While that may be true, (and we'll talk more about binders shortly), the last thing we want to do is stir up heavy metals unless we have all our ducks in a row.

Detoxification is like a puzzle. Your liver, kidneys, skin, lungs, lymphatic system, and digestive system are all pieces of that puzzle. Make no mistake, everything that passes your lips, be it a liquid, pill, or food, has an impact on the way those pieces fit together.

All things being equal, it's now time to *gently* prepare the body (that's you) for the first phase of detoxification.

THE 5'p.S. OF PREPARATION

To do this right, we would do well to remember the rule of 5'p.S. (proper planning prevents poor performance). Depending on your level of toxicity, this period of preparation may need to last anywhere from a few weeks to a few months.

Because you are such a wonderful and unique individual, there is no one size fits all approach.

The aim of this chapter is simple, it's helping remove known stressors from the body. The fewer things your body has to deal with, the better your chances of a successful outcome. Stressors are categorized into three main areas, physical, chemical, and emotional.

PHYSICAL STRESS

A physical stressor is an underlying injury that has been left unresolved. For example: if your arm is currently hanging off, then it's probably *not* the best time to send your body into detoxification mode. But not all physical stressors are so obvious or dramatic.

Stressors can be anything from an ongoing tooth infection to an open cut that hasn't had time to heal. For those looking for an alternative to antibiotics, Argentyn 23 (a bio-active silver hydrosol) can help fight lingering infections. And while antibiotics have a place, overuse will almost certainly disrupt your gut bacteria.

Antibiotics work by killing bacteria indiscriminately. When good and bad bacteria are treated as one, it's the equivalent of carpet bombing an area. Once the bacteria in the gut are disrupted, candida can get a pretty firm foothold. When left unchecked, candida will drill into the walls of your intestines. Once the delicate lining is damaged, we can then expect to see symptoms of leaky gut. And yup, leaky gut is another physical stressor.

Leaky gut is remarkably common in people dealing with both heavy metals and mold toxicity issues. Not least because vital nutrients are poorly absorbed. Without the right amount of nutrients, detoxification is disrupted. If this is you, don't panic. I'm aware that this is an important topic and I've dedicated the next chapter to it.

While we are on the subject, poor digestive health can also lead to inflammation. Acute, chronic, and systemic inflammation has been linked to just about every illness known to man! As I'm sure you already know, inflammation can occur anywhere in the body. It can linger silently like a smoldering fire, or it can be present wherever there is pain.

One day, I'd like to write a whole other book on the topic of inflammation, but for now, here's the main takeaway message: **Chronic inflammation will impair your ability to detoxify.** You know your own body better than I do. I'm simply suggesting that you get these things in order BEFORE diving headfirst into any detox protocol.

EMOTIONAL STRESS

By modern standards, emotional stress has become the new normal. Work, family, relationships are all significant sources of stress. Throw into the mix a boss or a landlord that's a jerk and stress can soon become relentless. Look, I get it, I really do, we all have problems. Some of these problems are out of our control and some are not. Either way, **your ability to detoxify takes a back seat every time you become overly stressed.**

Timing is everything in this life. If you are in the middle of moving to a new house, or your teenager just walked through the door with a triple nipple piercing, then perhaps now isn't the best time to detox your body. On the flip side, we detoxify best when we are resting or digesting.

Some of us manage stress better than others. If you are in the "others" camp, then an adaptogenic herb by the name of Ashwagandha may prove helpful. Some folks turn to alcohol as a way of coping which not only taxes the liver, it also leads us nicely to our next section – chemical stress.

CHEMICAL STRESS

Chemical stress refers to things like excessive alcohol intake, smoking, toxic cleaning products, over-the-counter medications, poor diet (hello again), recreational drugs, etc.

Mold also falls into this category. This is important, as an ongoing mold issue creates the very thing we are trying to avoid—a bottleneck! So, take a critical look around at your environment, now ask yourself, are any of these things making you sick, or are they keeping you sick?

If you are living in a stressful state, I'd bet the farm (if I had one) that your magnesium levels are almost depleted. Magnesium has a nourishing effect on the nervous system. That said, not all magnesium is made equal and as mentioned in the previous chapter, many supplement forms of magnesium are poorly absorbed in the gut. Here's a neat way to bypass this problem ...

You can boost your magnesium levels by transdermal means. This simply means it's absorbed through the skin rather than the gut. There are lots of magnesium sprays on the market but the one I like best is *EASE* by Activation Products. It's super easy to use, you simply spray it directly onto your skin. Magnesium is a WIN/WIN, as it helps with a bunch of things. It's also a cofactor in more than 300 enzyme systems that regulate diverse biochemical reactions in the body! But most importantly, magnesium is an important mineral because it makes you feel good while also helping the body to detoxify.

REMINERALIZE

Minerals are the game changers in detoxification. Without minerals, our detox wheels will be spinning, but we won't be able to pull out of the garage. That said, you can't just pop mineral pills thinking you have covered all the bases. This will surely tax the liver and kidneys, a much better way to increase minerals is by cleaning up your diet.

You can do this by eating *less* processed foods (I know right, that old chestnut) while at the same time cranking up nutrient-dense foods.

It's often said that a healthy diet is the cornerstone of good health. But unless you have a firm understanding of toxicity, the health benefits of nutrition are sometimes lost. Lest we forget, organic food is tested for pesticides, *not* heavy metals.

Having an abundance of minerals in your body helps to smooth out any detox bumps in the road. Fortunately, increasing your mineral count is relatively easy and inexpensive to do.

Any vegetables that have the same color running through them will be naturally higher in nutrients. Think beets, carrots, etc. You can also take some of the workloads off your digestive system by turning these vegetables into liquid (AKA juicing). But your ability to absorb those nutrients largely depends on the integrity of your gut lining. You can improve the integrity of your gut lining with bone broth. Bone broth is an ideal choice, as it's also rich in minerals.

You can add more minerals to your diet through natural sea salt. (Although some sea salts contain more minerals than others). I've found **Baja Gold Sea Salt** to be a pretty decent brand that's produced from the mineral-rich Sea of Cortez. I've also read good things about **Celtic Sea Salt,** which you can find in your local supermarket. At a pinch (pun intended), Himalayan salt also works, but some of the cheaper brands can be high in contaminants. Either way, it's a huge improvement over regular table salt which belongs in the trash can. As a side note, you can also add a little mineral-rich salt to your morning coffee. When it comes to increasing minerals, we also make sure we get enough selenium, *here's why...*

SELENIUM

Selenium is a mineral found in soil, water, and some foods. If you eat fish (or fish products) selenium makes you *less* susceptible to the effects of methylmercury. On the flip side, we could argue that when there's not enough selenium in your diet, you are *more* susceptible to the effects of methylmercury. *Hmm. I see.*

Selenium helps to protect the body from free radicals, it's also a cofactor to glutathione peroxidase (more on glutathione coming shortly). Selenium supports a strong immune system and helps to regulate thyroid function. A selenium deficiency is sometimes linked to thyroid conditions such as Hashimoto's thyroiditis. Brazil Nuts are an excellent source of selenium. Each Brazil nut is said to contain between 50–75 mcg. You can also take selenium in supplement form, although it's best taken with Vitamin E.

As a side note: Once opened, Vitamin E is best stored in the fridge to prevent it from going rancid.

BEET JUICE IS HARD TO BEAT

As we learned earlier, the liver is a key player in detoxification. You can support the liver by drinking a small amount of beet juice first thing in the morning on an empty stomach. Beet juice aids digestion, it also lowers blood pressure and serves as a natural blood cleanser. Beet juice contains betaine, a substance known to prevent or reduce fatty deposits in the liver. A starting dose of one fluid ounce every morning for the first week, followed by two ounces the second week can prove helpful.

That said, beet juice isn't recommended for everyone. Beets are naturally high in oxalates, which should be avoided by anyone with suspected kidney stones. If this is you, switch to drinking freshly squeezed lemon juice diluted in twelve ounces of filtered water. Doing this first thing in the morning will also help cleanse the liver.

WHY BROCCOLI IS A SUPER SPROUT.

Broccoli sprouts are a great addition to your diet. They provide a source of glucoraphanin which is then converted to sulforaphane. We'll cover this in more detail later, for now, just remember that broccoli sprouts help the body to detoxify more efficiently. You can buy broccoli sprouts directly from the supermarket, but they are easy to grow in a Mason jar. This is known as "Sprouting." It offers peak nutrition for pennies on the dollar (and you don't even need a garden). A simple google search will show you just how easy sprouting is.

Before we leave this section, be sure to add fermented foods to your diet, these will help with your immune system. Last but not least, be sure to get your daily dose of the morning sunshine.

Sunshine is the best way to get your vitamin d levels up. Vitamin D supports the body during detoxification.

Next, we'll look at ways to absorb more of those important nutrients through your digestive system. Good digestion is the key to detoxification.

Chapter 7: IT TAKES GUTS TO LEAK

Jean Anthelme Brillat-Savarin once said, "Tell me what you eat, and I will tell you what you are." Today, that statement would be more accurate if it read "Tell me what you *absorb,* and I will tell you what you are."

In this chapter, I'll highlight some of the problems caused by poor absorption, and then I'll offer some simple solutions. That said, if you are experiencing ongoing digestive issues, it's worth getting yourself checked out by an "informed" healthcare provider. Sadly, the mere mention of a leaky gut in your average physician's office can result in an uncomfortably long stare. As you may have guessed, leaky gut is still medically classified as a theory. Ever wonder why?

Well, the short answer is clinical trials cost money. Nutrition just isn't sexy enough to pay for million-dollar trials. Alas, any attempt to medicate our way out of a poor diet displays poor judgment. And while most doctors agree that damage to the intestinal lining is plausible. Few seem willing to accept that it causes a cascade of other health issues.

Here's a visual representation of the problem.

In your mind's eye, imagine holding a bicycle inner tube. Next, take a pair of scissors and cut the tube so that it hangs down in a single straight line. Then place the tube on the floor in front of you. What you now have is a design very similar to your digestive system. Both are hollow tubes with an opening at the top (the mouth) and an exit at the bottom (anus).

If we now forced food into the top of the inner tube and squeezed it down to the bottom, sooner or later, food would exit at the bottom. Crudely, this is how the body expels waste.

Now hold that image, got it?

If we again pick up those imaginary scissors. Only this time, make several microscopic nicks to the inner tube (anywhere you like). And if we stuff imaginary food down into the tube, small particles will soon be oozing out of those tiny nicks. In the body, this is how tiny food particles find their way into the bloodstream.

That's not good, right?

Not really. Your immune system is smart, but it isn't expecting to see food floating around in the bloodstream, or even worse, bits of fecal matter (ew gross). As far as the immune system is concerned, all bacon sandwich particles are safely trapped inside the inner tube (AKA your digestive tract).

When the immune system spots something it doesn't recognize, it gets a little freaked out. Once that happens, the whole system flies into a code red alert. Throw into the mix a few gallons of glyphosate and Boomshakalaka! Say hello to food sensitivities and your new best friend chronic inflammation. But our intestines aren't meant to leak, so why would they do this to us?

As mentioned earlier, candida can be a contributing factor. But so can proteins, which are found in gluten. These proteins are notoriously difficult to break down, more so when they are grown in contaminated soil. This isn't rocket science. When the gut is continually damaged, it becomes permeable.

Let's explore this concept a little, I'll then show you a couple of things that can help resolve a leaky gut.

From the moment we swallow it, to the time it leaves the body, food is meant to stay *inside* the digestive system. It's both unusual and unnatural for food to wander into the bloodstream. Some might say that it's almost as unnatural as the way we now grow our food.

Let's simplify. The foods we eat will either deplete our body's mineral supply or it will replenish it. And yet, the standard western diet relies heavily on grains. Most of which have been "modified" or soaked in Roundup to increase crop yields. While an increase in crops sounds good in theory, nobody knows for sure how this will impact us long term. I'm just going to leave this next statement hanging while it sinks in.

Food has changed more in the last fifty years than it has in the previous 10,000 years!

For many, the gluten found in wheat, barley, and rye is already causing a wide range of reactions. These reactions can range from a feeling of general fatigue to mental confusion. Add into the mix a few hundred food additives and we shouldn't be all that surprised when people struggle to detoxify.

Adding to the problem, most of our food is now sprayed with some pretty heavy-duty pesticides. This has become an everyday farming practice and nobody seems to mind. Many of these pesticides contain EDCs (endocrine-disrupting chemicals). They work by disrupting the central nervous systems of bugs. And get this, some of the newer insecticides work by exploding the insect's gut. *Hmm, I see.*

GLUTEN-FREE? - Not so fast.

Once grains become a problem, switching to "gluten-free" products is unlikely to solve the problem. Think of a smoker switching to a different brand of cigarettes as a way of limiting symptoms. *So, what's the answer?*

Once your immune system reacts to gluten, the only viable solution is to go grain-free. The good news is this is easy to do. Simply stop buying man-made foods that come in a box, a can, or a packet and replace them with whole foods. We could make this sound more complicated if you like. But it's probably best if you just think of it this way … if the food comes from a manufacturing plant, don't eat it. If it comes from a plant, you are good to go.

Ironically, the cleanest foods *aren't* always sitting in the organic section of your supermarket. Lest we forget, the average vegetable travels 1500 miles to get to your dinner plate. With that in mind, you might find a better deal at your local farmer's market.

My book titled "<u>The Healing Point</u>" has more tips on health and nutrition.

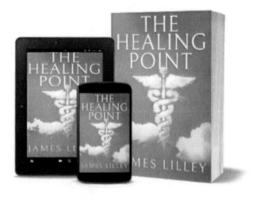

It's like the Swiss Army knife of health books. If it's not in here, you'll probably never need it.

S.O.S ... I STILL NEED TO FIX MY GUT

It's no secret that your gut is pivotal to your overall health. Avoiding foods that are known to irritate the gut lining is a given, but is there anything else we can do to help the healing process? *As it happens, you are in luck!*

Combining colostrum, bone broth, and a high-quality probiotic can help speed up repairs to the gut lining. These three bad boys work synergistically, but as always, the devil is in the details. Not all colostrum/bone broth/probiotics are made equal. Fortunately, I've done some research in this area and below are the brands I think you will find helpful. That said, it's your personal choice, you can substitute any of these brands. I'm simply trying to save you some time.

Colostrum: Sold by Mt Capra

Bone Broth: Sold by Kettle and Fire (Or make your own, it's pretty easy to do)

Probiotics: Sold by Seed

For best results, take these in the morning on an empty stomach. If you are on a tight budget, try supplementing with L-glutamine instead. The recommended dose will be on the label.

All things being equal, the biggest problem after leaky gut is poor quality stomach acid. Some might say the two go hand in hand. Hold that thought because this important topic is covered in the following chapter.

Chapter 8: STOMACH ACID IS STRONG FOR A REASON

Hopefully, you are beginning to see that detoxification is a step-by-step process. But if any of the steps are missing, then results will be lackluster at best. These steps could be thought of as a combination lock. And unless ALL of the numbers are correctly lined up, the lock isn't going to open.

In this chapter, we'll be looking a little deeper into your stomach acid. **This topic is often overlooked, but it's one of the most important in the book.** Strong stomach acid plays a huge role in protecting us from harmful bacteria that are sometimes ingested with food. Trust me, if your stomach acid is out of kilter, then EVERYTHING else is out.

Normally, the acid in your stomach is so strong that it can dissolve metal. I know what you're thinking because I thought. If the acid can dissolve metal, then why doesn't it burn right through the lining of the stomach? That's a great question and before we get to the answer, we need to back up a little.

Digestion begins in the mouth. The more times you chew your food the less work your stomach acid has to do. If it helps, think of it this way, the better you chew, the better you poo! After chewing, food is then swallowed, and it travels down a long tube called the esophagus. At the end of that tube is a small muscular valve that opens up just enough to allow the food to drop into a bath of stomach acid. *But wait, there's a problem. Can you see it?*

Whatever it was we just ate, now needs to be broken down into a form of liquid mush. This helps with absorption as it moves through the intestine. Food doesn't turn to mush on its own, it needs the help of stomach acid (also known as hydrochloric acid, or HCL).

The acid in your stomach has been working this way since the beginning of time, and you have to marvel at the design. Food drops down the shoot into a bath of acid—splosh! The acid then turns food into liquid mush; this mush then oozes out a little at a time into the small intestine. So far so good, right? *Meh, not so fast...*

What if the stomach acid has become weak through illness, neglect, medications, abuse, or chemotherapy? All of these things can reduce stomach acid.

The *entire* process of digestion hinges on this pivotal stage. If the acid isn't strong enough, a whole chain reaction of negative events begins to unfold. Not least, all those valuable nutrients will struggle to be fully absorbed. We need those nutrients to help us detoxify and to rebuild our cells.

HEARTBURN—A BILLION DOLLAR INDUSTRY

Bloating, belching, flatulence, indigestion, diarrhea, and constipation are all clues that something isn't quite right with the stomach. In some circumstances, a person with weak stomach acid may also suffer from heartburn. *Wait a second, did you catch that?*

But isn't heartburn treated by the million-dollar antacid industry? *If only it were that simple.*

If this is you, how have years of taking antacids been working for you? Has it fixed the problem, or does it just keep coming back, again and again, and again?

I'd like to suggest that antacids add to the problem by making already low stomach acid even lower. The stomach strives to balance itself out, but it cannot correct the problem with a belly full of alkaline pills. Obviously, if you are taking a prescription antacid, this is something you need to work that out with your doctor. While you are there, it might be worth getting tested for H-pylori, which is a type of bacteria known to reduce stomach acid.

Sometimes, we simply have to get out of the way and let the stomach do the job it was designed to do, which is making acid strong enough to dissolve metal!

So why would low stomach acid give some folks heartburn?

At the end of the esophagus there's a kind of valve. It's known as the Lower Esophageal Sphincter (or LES), it's really a muscle that contracts much the same way the anus does. Its job is to form a tight seal to stop acid from slipping back up into the esophagus (where it can cause damage and heartburn).

Some schools of thought suggest that the LES valve has some degree of sensitivity to the acid in the stomach. When the stomach acid is too low, it may be fooled into opening back up. Hence, all those antacids really aren't helping. If this is you, and you have been on the merry-go-round for any length of time, then perhaps it may be worth trying a different approach.

For now, the problem is much bigger than heartburn. Weak stomach acid has a domino effect throughout the remaining stages of digestion. That liquid mush (the fancy name for it is chyme or chymus) now becomes a semi-fluid mass of partly digested food. It's then expelled by the stomach into the duodenum. *Say what now?*

Without wanting to confuse you with lots of fancy names let's just work with the primary rule of physics and say that all shit rolls downhill. As it does so, the chime (AKA liquid mush) passes a bunch of important sensory checkpoints on the way down. These checkpoints scrutinize the quality of the mush.

In theory, if the quality of the stomach acid is good, so is the quality of the liquid mush. If not, then it's a case of too bad, so sad, because when it comes to poop, there's no turning back.

Okay, let's pause here for a second.

Before I'm accused of turning the topic of digestion into a crude oversimplification, perhaps I should point out that the research I do on these subjects is often as intense as it is mind-numbing. I'm simply looking to spare you that ordeal by making this information enjoyable to read. So, with your permission, may I press on using nonmedical terms like poop and liquid mush?

"If you can't explain it simply you don't understand it well enough" - Albert Einstein

Okay, once our liquid mush enters the small intestine, enzymes are eagerly waiting to break things down even more. Obviously, this presents a problem if the hydrochloric acid in the stomach isn't strong enough to do its job properly.

NOW IT GETS TRICKY

There are three main enzymes the body uses to aid in digestion. These are amylase, protease, and lipase, but there are also a few specialized enzymes that help in the process too. Cells that line the intestines also make enzymes called maltase, sucrase, and lactase, and each can convert a specific type of sugar into glucose. Do we need to know all these terms as a layperson? *Probably not, but I know medical student types worry when I use terms like liquid mush.*

Two more enzymes by the names of renin and gelatinase then come into play. Renin acts on proteins in milk, converting them into smaller molecules called peptides. These are then fully digested by pepsin. *I know right, who thinks like this?*

But wait, there's more!

Gelatinase digests gelatin and collagen—two large proteins in meat—into moderately sized compounds whose digestion is then completed by pepsin, trypsin, and chymotrypsin, producing amino acids.

Just saying ... isn't it easier to just say "certain enzymes help us absorb our nutrients," I think so.

Either way, if weak stomach acid allows partially undigested food to move through the digestive system, the whole delicate balance is disrupted. A domino effect then occurs as the liver, gallbladder, and pancreas also pick up on the lack of acidity and react accordingly. If weak acid in the stomach isn't doing its job optimally, it's a safe bet that neither is anything else.

Rather than trying to bolt the stable door after the horse has fled, it may be helpful to increase stomach acid rather than decrease it.

RECAP

We need strong stomach acid to help us break down our foods, especially proteins. Strong stomach acid also helps kill off any harmful bacteria that can enter with food. Weak stomach acid, on the other hand, can cause a whole host of health problems.

At this point, you should now realize the importance of your stomach acid. How helpful would it be if there was a simple test you could do from home to check your stomach acid? *Hold on to your hat, there's one below!*

STOMACH ACID TEST

1. First thing in the morning, mix 1/4 teaspoon of baking soda in 4–6 ounces of room temp water.

2. Drink the baking soda on an empty stomach.

3. Time how long it takes before you belch.

4. If you have not belched within five minutes, stop timing.

If your stomach is producing adequate amounts of stomach acid, you'll likely belch within two to three minutes. Early and repeated belching may be due to excessive stomach acid. But don't confuse these burps with small little burps from swallowing air while drinking the solution). Any belching after three minutes indicates a low acid level.

Keep in mind that this test is only a basic indicator. You might want to do more follow up testing with your primary caregiver to determine the level of your stomach acid.

This test is also not considered accurate enough to rule out low stomach acid. To rule out low stomach acid, you will need to ask your doctor to conduct a Heidelberg test or Betaine HCL challenge test.

HOW TO FIX LOW STOMACH ACID

If stomach acid is found to be too low, there are lots of ways to increase it. One way is to supplement with Betaine HCL, (which is best taken with protein).

Another is to take a tablespoon of apple cider vinegar (ACV) ten minutes before each meal. To help increase stomach acid, simply mix the ACV in 8 oz. of room temp water and drink (for health, not taste).

If ACV isn't your thing, then try mixing one freshly squeezed lemon, 4 oz. of water, approximately three knuckles of chopped raw ginger, and a half teaspoon of sea salt. Leave this mixture to pickle for a few days and then take one teaspoon of the mixture before meals. It's an acquired taste, but if your stomach acid is low, your body will begin to crave it. As with anything new, start with a small test dose and go slow.

If you only take one thing away from this book, then let it be the value of your stomach acid. Putting our health back together is a process. And slowly, piece by piece, we are now bringing all the pieces of the detoxification puzzle into view.

Finally, if you were still wondering how stomach acid can dissolve metal, but it doesn't burn through the stomach, then here's your answer. The stomach has a mucous membrane. It's a wall of snotty cells that are constantly replaced; as one-layer burns through, another layer steps in to replace it.

Chapter 9: OPENING CLOSED DETOX DOORS

In a very short space of time, we have covered quite a lot of ground together. Let's quickly recap.

First and foremost, we identified what heavy metals are and how to reduce your exposure to them. We then talked about the importance of testing and the various options open to you. We've also covered the six main pathways that your body uses to expel toxins, and what you can do to help them.

We've discussed the importance of sleep and how to do it right. We've uncovered the physical, chemical, and emotional stressors that prevent the body from detoxifying. We looked at minerals and how poor absorption of them will have an impact on your overall health. We've looked at stomach acid and why it's the key to good digestion. *Phew, that's quite a list and the best bits are still to come!*

Let's take a look at how toxins move around the body. From here I'll be using the term "toxins" in the broadest sense of the word. I'm applying it to cover *anything* that's considered harmful to your health.

Toxins travel to the liver and kidneys. They do this in two ways, either through the blood or through the lymph. *Let's break this process down a little.*

When blood filters through the liver, it sends toxins out to the Gastrointestinal tract. The GI tract then sends whatever it doesn't like the look of to the toilet bowl. *Hoorah, for good digestion!*

The kidneys also play a role in filtering blood. Anything they don't like is then sent to the urinary tract, and from there, it once again meets the toilet bowl. *Hoorah, for sanitation!*

This next step is logical, and it's one that most well-meaning health gurus get wrong. Having covered so much ground together, most are now keen to begin removing all those toxins hiding in our fat cells. *But now there's just one teeny-weeny problem to worry about. Can you see it?*

If you are reading books on detoxification, then I'll assume that you probably have your fair share of toxins flowing through your blood and lymph. Adding more to your burden would almost certainly guarantee us first place in the crash and burn competition. This is often referred to as a Herxheimer reaction" or a "healing crisis". A more critical mind might refer to it as poor planning. *Here's why...*

Imagine a garbage truck coming down the road to pick up your trash. But as the truck gets closer, you see it's already full. Yes, you could try to squeeze your bag of trash onto the truck, but as it drives away, we shouldn't be surprised if it then spills out onto the floor. The ideal solution is to wait for the driver to return with an empty truck. Lo-and-behold, when it comes to detoxification, if we empty our proverbial garbage truck first, then the healing "crisis" magically goes away.

Let's start by how *not* to do this.

When the body already has too many toxins already circulating in the blood and lymph, throwing detox supplements at the problem isn't helping. It's the equivalent of the trash falling out of the truck. When the liver can't cope, it will simply send toxins straight back into the bloodstream. Can we now say hello to fatigue, headache, and anxiety? *I think so.*

Here's the deal. Before attempting to pull toxins out of fat cells, toxins circulating in the bloodstream must be cleaned up first. In effect, we are emptying our garbage truck.

WHY STRESS MAKES A MESS

At this point, let's remind ourselves that the body doesn't do a lot of detoxifying when it's in a stressed state. If there's a Bengal tiger loose in your back garden, toxins *aren't* going to leave the bloodstream if your body feels threatened in any way.

Here's why.

Our ancestors knew when to fight and when to run. And when either option is applied, the whole detoxification process shuts down. This is commonly known as the fight-or-flight response, and it's controlled by the **sympathetic nervous system.** When this bad boy kicks in, your body is firmly locked in "oh shit mode." It's making split-second choices to either fight the dragon or carry you as far away from the dragon as your hairy little legs will take you.

When the body is in this stressed state, the detox doors stay firmly closed and it doesn't matter how much cilantro your well-meaning health guru shakes at the problem. Lest we forget, stress comes at us in many forms. Unless your favorite pastime is experiencing detox symptoms, then stirring up a body full of toxins while you are in a sympathetic state is simply foolhardy.

Fortunately, the detox doors become WIDE OPEN for business once the danger passes. This is where your **parasympathetic nervous system** now kicks in. It's your chill out button, the same button that helps us go to sleep. Or if you prefer, it's the rest and digest state.

Stressful situations can come and go daily. One of the fastest, most effective ways to bring ourselves back into a relaxed parasympathetic state is with deep breathing exercises. I know that sounds a tad "woo-woo" but trust me, it's absolutely true! We still have a lot to cover so if it's all the same to you, feel free to check out a few YouTube videos on deep breathing exercises. You can crank this up a notch by combining deep breathing exercises with CBD oil.

Now that we have an understanding of the rest and digest stage let's bring our garbage truck back around. Remember, at this stage, we aren't looking to pull toxins and heavy metals out of fat cells, we are simply looking to drain off what's already circulating in the bloodstream and lymph.

To help us do this, it's important to have all of our other detox ducks nicely in a row, hence, all the steps leading up to this point have been moving us in this direction. If for any reason you still aren't sure what they are, simply go back and read through this book again. *I won't even charge you an extra penny for doing so.*

Okay, whenever an attempt is made to remove toxins from the body, what's the golden rule? Let me hear it … **don't be greedy!** This means heavy metals must be removed slowly.

DRAINAGE AND BILE

It might surprise you to know that the key to all of this is your tongue. When the tongue senses bitter flavors it opens up the gallbladder, which in turn releases bile. Bile is a greenish-brown alkaline fluid that aids digestion. It's secreted by the liver but is essentially stored in the gallbladder. Bile helps us to digest fatty foods. In its most basic form, think of it as the dishwasher liquid removing grease from after dinner plates. *Why is this important to know?*

When we aren't moving bile, we aren't moving toxins or if you like, it's the same transporters that remove bile also move toxins.

There are lots of bitters you can ingest to increase bile. Earlier, we mentioned dandelion, which is a bitter herb. You can also eat dandelion leaves straight from your garden. If that's a little too crunchy for ya, (hey I'm not judging) then you could always add freshly squeezed lemon juice to a glass of water. For best results, drink it first thing in the morning on an empty stomach. Milk thistle is a wonderful bitter that gently helps to clean the liver. You can also take it with lemon water.

I don't want to overwhelm you with information, but as you become more experienced, you may find it helpful to try a blend of bitter herbs. A local herbalist is a good person to help you with this. An herbalist may also suggest burdock, which can help clean the blood.

When bitters are taken twenty minutes before a meal, they help to get the digestive juices flowing. This includes our old friend stomach acid (AKA hydrochloric acid). This is where all this now begins to fit neatly together.

Hitting the drainage button with bitters ensures that all those circulating toxins are now moving nicely along to our two main detoxification pathways—the liver and kidneys.

And here's where it gets interesting.

With the detox doors open (we are in rest and digest mode) adding a few natural diuretics such as green tea, dandelion (hello again), goldenrod, etc. can help to flush out impurities from the bladder and kidneys. It's the equivalent of turning on the faucet to the sink.

We can also turn up the bile dial with a little help from phosphatidylcholine. Phosphatidylcholine (also known as PC) is a ubiquitous, naturally occurring phospholipid molecule. *I know right, what the heck does that mean?*

Phosphatidylcholine is naturally found in the body. It can also be found in (free-range) eggs, soybeans, mustard, sunflower, and other foods. The term "phosphatidylcholine" is sometimes used interchangeably with "lecithin," although the two are closely related, they are not exactly the same.

A component of phosphatidylcholine is choline. Choline is important for liver function and brain development. Choline is a precursor to the neurotransmitter acetylcholine, which opens a protein channel, stimulating muscle contraction. We could quite easily take ourselves down a phosphatidylcholine rabbit hole here, but for now, it's worth noting that a choline deficiency can contribute to the development of nonalcoholic fatty liver disease. Millions of people have a fatty liver, and most won't even realize it. This sounds good right up until it morphs into something more serious such as cirrhosis of the liver or even liver failure. *Hmm, I see, said the blind man.*

The trick to reversing a nonalcoholic fatty liver is to treat it early. This can be done by reducing the toxic burden on your liver, eating a balanced diet, getting plenty of exercise, and using the right supplementation.

When it comes to supplementation, a little common sense will serve you better than going to the problem with guns blazing. Whenever you try something new, first check with your primary health caregiver, and then start with a small dose and go slow. Taking a few well-targeted supplements is like using a sniper rifle to pick off toxins in the body. Taking too many, too quickly, is taking the shotgun approach. Given that the body likes to be in balance, which approach is going to give you better results?

Think of it this way, we all need oxygen to survive. But as any scuba diver will tell you, too much oxygen can result in convulsions, pulmonary barotrauma, and death! Too much of anything is a bad thing. We all need water to survive, but the downside of too much water is called drowning! Keep these examples in mind as we cover our final chapters.

Bottom line: Diuretics help us to pee more, which drains any excess fluid through the kidneys and urinary system. To compensate for this, it's important to be drinking enough water. Bitters stimulate bile, which plays a key role in moving toxins through the GI tract.

Like what you read so far? A short review from you would be awesome!

Chapter: 10: BURLY BINDERS

Imagine yourself at a busy night club and the person heading towards you is a known troublemaker. He's been barred from the club several times in the past, but somehow, he always manages to sneak back in. He does this by blending in with a sea of other people. Fortunately, there's a burly bouncer on duty who's just spotted him.

Before the troublemaker has a chance to cause you (or your glow-stick) any problems, the bouncer picks him up by the scruff of his neck. He then frog-marches him to the nearest exit. No matter how much the troublemaker struggles, the bouncer isn't letting go of him. At least until he's well and truly thrown out of the exit door. *Good riddance to bad news!*

In this analogy, think of the busy nightclub as your GI tract. A lot is going on and not all of it is good. The troublemaker that keeps coming back is our toxic heavy metal. As for the burly bouncer, he's playing the role of a binder.

Binders latch onto heavy metals and refuse to let them go until they reach the body's exit door. One flush of the toilet and your toxic burden has just been lowered. *Hoorah!*

But without a binder, heavy metals moving through the GI tract are quickly reabsorbed into the bloodstream. It's the equivalent of the bouncer throwing someone out only to have them sneak back into via the side door.

There are lots of binders on the market. In this chapter, we'll look at six of them. As you read through this list, keep in mind that some folks are more toxic than others. When it comes to binders, you may need a little more, or you may need a lot less. It all depends on where you are at and with your health. In most cases, a little tinkering may be required to find your sweet spot. Either way, when you take a binder it's super important to stay hydrated. *Here's why ...*

Binders need to be flushed through the system and water helps to do this. Without wanting to sound like a broken record, the trick to getting this right is to start with a small binder dose and go slow. You can always add a little later, but it's not so easy to take it away. The body works best when opposing forces or influences are balanced. This is sometimes referred to as being in a state of equilibrium. In plain English, this simply means that all things in the body (that's you) are a delicate balancing act.

Okay, without further ado. Let's kick off with our first binder, which is activated charcoal, for no other reason other than my tiny OCD brain likes to do things in alphabetical order.

#1 ACTIVATED CHARCOAL

Activated charcoal is a manufactured product, which means you won't find it naturally in foods. Making activated charcoal involves heating carbon-rich materials, such as wood, peat, or coconut shells to a very high temperature. Activated charcoal then becomes an extremely adsorbent fine black powder. Once ingested, it will bind to molecules, ions, atoms, etc.

But what the heck does that even mean?

Activated charcoal carries a slight negative electrical charge. This negative charge acts like a magnet seeking out positively charged toxins. *Wait a second, I thought all positive things were supposed to be good?*

Nope, in this case, it's all flipped. "Negative ions" are good, and "positive ions" are what make us feel crappy. *Here's an example...*

The highest concentrations of negative ions are found outside in nature. They are abundant with waterfalls, on mountain tops, in forests, and next to the ocean. Think back to the last time you had your toes in the water, how did you feel? Recharged, energized?

Now, by comparison, imagine standing in a crowded, stuffy room full of people. Does it make you feel like running outside screaming, "I need my lungs filled with oxygen?" Me too, I'm weird like that. It's all to do with a *lack* of negative ions in the air.

Negative ions enhance immune function, purify the blood, and help revitalize cell metabolism. They also help to neutralize free radicals that cause us to age. Who knew breathing fresh air was so important?

Any idea where you can find an abundance of unhealthy, positive ions? Top marks if you said:

polluted cities, crowded bars, industrial areas, and confined spaces such as stuffy offices. It's all to do with the fact positive ions are molecules that have lost one or more electrons. *Too bad, so sad.*

Now that we have that housework out of the way, let's get back to our main topic, which is binders.

Activated charcoal is so effective at being a binder that emergency rooms use it to treat overdoses. Keep this in mind as it can have an impact on prescription medications. When in doubt, always check with your primary caregiver.

Activated charcoal has a long history dating back thousands of years. Ancient Egyptians used it to overcome food poisoning. And in 1831, the French Academy of Medicine reported that a man by the name of Tovery used it to survive a lethal dose of strychnine! It was claimed that he managed to do this by swallowing a large dose of activated charcoal. Personally, I wouldn't try this one at home, but it does highlight the remarkable binding ability of activated charcoal.

Activated charcoal is sometimes found in natural toothpaste, it's also used in water filters, and some people use it in the fridge to absorb toxic smells. Activated charcoal is sometimes used to extract moisture from the air. As versatile as this binder is, it's not something you want to take long term.

How come?

Activated charcoal has a dark side. It is so effective that it can bind to important minerals, vitamins, and antioxidants found in food. Over time, this can deplete the body of good things it needs. Hence, you wouldn't want to take it day in, day out. As with most things, moderation is key. It pays to take periodic breaks from any substance that binds this well.

However, if you get a sudden bellyache, activated charcoal can be a godsend. This is good to know if you find yourself on vacation in some sketchy corner of the world. Activated will also treat hangovers. *Hey, I ain't judging. I'm just sitting here thinking about all the ways we mistreat the liver.*

#2 BENTONITE CLAY

Bentonite Clay has been used for centuries to pull out toxins from the body. As with anything that stands the test of time, it's usually for good reason. When bentonite clay is mixed with water, the molecular components change and it produces a slight electrical charge. This negative charge attracts positively charged toxins. In the GI tract, it works like a magnetic sponge.

Bentonite clay is also pretty good at removing a wide range of stomach bugs hence, it can be helpful with diarrhea. If this is you, a quarter teaspoon of bentonite clay in a glass of warm water may help. It looks like a cup of mud, but despite this, it's actually surprisingly easy to drink. You can also add it to food which doesn't taste great but for some, it can be a better way to take it.

#3 CHLORELLA

Chlorella is a genus of single-celled green algae belonging to the division Chlorophyta. If that made no sense to you let's try this. In the gut, chlorella likes to bind to mercury and lead. That said, not all chlorella is made equal. There is good quality chlorella out there while others are worthless junk. As with most things, you tend to get what you pay for. You'll want to find a "broken cell wall chlorella." Personally, I like Chlorella Pyrenoidosa which is sold by Biopure.

Chlorella is a waterborne organism with a high concentration of chlorophyll. Chlorophyll gives all living plants its green pigment. Chlorella is super rich with phytonutrients, amino acids, chlorophyll, beta-carotene, potassium, phosphorus, biotin, magnesium, and B-complex vitamins.

To help you understand the importance of Chlorella, here's a short, one-minute video clip from Dr. Klinghardt (who happens to know a thing or two when it comes to detoxification). https://www.youtube.com/watch?v=RG_6zn1XEbw

BLENDING OUR ABC's

It's worth noting, results are sometimes enhanced by blending activated charcoal with bentonite clay, and chlorella. Simply use an equal amount of each and mix them in a large glass of water. If you are using powdered forms, a conservative amount (for a relatively healthy adult) could be considered a quarter teaspoon. If you aren't sure, start with a smaller dose and work your way up. Mix it up well and continue drinking plenty of water to help flush those toxins out.

What's neat about blending these three is you are covering a lot of bases all at the same time. For example, activated charcoal goes after endotoxins (a toxin that is present inside a bacterial cell). Whereas Bentonite clay goes after aflatoxins (toxins produced by certain molds). This leaves chlorella free to mop up metals such as mercury. As a bonus, pesticides and herbicides are also being reduced at the same time.

#4 MODIFIED CITRUS PECTIN

Pectin is a naturally occurring substance found in berries, apples, and other fruit. I know what you are thinking because I had the same thought, why modify something that's already found naturally?

That's a great question, and the short answer is this allows parts of citrus fruits to be turned into a powder. During this process, molecules are made smaller so that they are more easily absorbed into your bloodstream. The result allows your body to benefit from more than just pectin's fibrous properties.

Some vendors claim that modified citrus pectin may help with prostate cancer. Others suggest it can be beneficial for cellular health. From our perspective, our interest is in its ability to remove heavy metals from the GI tract which it does well.

There are lots of options when it comes to buying modified citrus pectin, but one of the most studied is PectaSol-C sold by ecoNugenics.

#5 IMD (Intestinal Metal Detox)

IMD is a highly purified silica with covalently bonded elements. This simply means IMD binds to heavy metals such as mercury in the gut. IMD comes in powdered form and does not contain any known allergens or fillers. IMD is more expensive than other binders, as it's much stronger. As such, it's best taken under the advice of a health care practitioner.

IMD is usually only taken for five days at a time and then backed away from it for two days. Given that it can take years for metals to build up in your body, you can expect to be chipping away at this stage for several months.

#6 ZEOLITES

Zeolites can be produced industrially, and they can be naturally occurring. The latter forms where volcanic rock and ash finds alkaline groundwater. A honeycomb structure is then formed, which carries a negative charge. This negative charge bonds to positively charged toxins that trap heavy metals, chemicals, and other volatile compounds inside the honeycomb. Unlike activated charcoal, zeolite does so without removing vital nutrients.

    This makes it a good entry point binder for the newbie detoxer. It's relatively inexpensive, and it works like a magnet trapping positively charged toxins such as lead, mercury, arsenic, and cadmium. This, in turn, helps to keep energy levels up and the immune system working at an optimal level. That said, not all zeolites are made equal and some pick contaminants during the formation process.

    You can find one of the better zeolites at https://detox101.thegoodinside.com/ It's a highly effective binder, and it's ALWAYS tested for purity.

Are there other binders that can pull junk out of your trunk? Yes, lots, but the aim of this chapter isn't to overwhelm you, it to provide you with enough information to get you started. Hope it helps.

Chapter 11: DETOXIFICATION UNLEASHED

It's no secret that when the body is overrun with toxins, the detoxification process begins to slow down. In some cases, it may even come to a grinding halt. With nowhere for toxic substances to go, the body takes a deep sigh, and then stores toxins in fat cells. It does this in an attempt to keep dangerous materials away from vital organs. At this point, weight gain and chronic fatigue become common complaints.

For some, the storing away of toxins such as heavy metals, toxic molds, PCBs, will continue until one day something finally gives way. The medical terms for this are "death and disease."

Reducing any further exposure to a known toxin is always a smart first step. But this alone is unlikely to clear the backlog. However, with the right approach, it is possible to remove years of toxins that have become lodged inside layers of fat. To help us do this, it's important to optimize glutathione levels. We can then tap into a remarkable pathway known as Nrf2. Before we get to that point, let us first explore what glutathione is and how it benefits us.

GLUTATHIONE

Glutathione (GSH) is a molecule found in the body. It consists of three amino acids being glutamic acid, cysteine, and glycine. When these bad boys get together, they form a formidable detoxifying gang. Between them, they are capable of riding the body of metals, molds, free radicals, etc.

A poor diet, underlying health conditions, and the natural aging process all decrease glutathione. A clear sign that your levels are running low is a poor immune function. This can make a person more prone to catching coughs and colds every year. Fortunately, there are ways to boost your levels back up.

When it comes to supplements, most are poorly absorbed in the gut. This makes them about as useful as a wooden frying pan. A better option is to take glutathione as a liposome (a little fat bubble that glutathione fits into). This helps glutathione survive the digestion process. You could also ask your doctor to administer glutathione intravenously. Before we hand responsibility over to anyone carrying a sharp needle, perhaps we should explore a smarter, less invasive option. What if I told you that your body could make its *own* high-quality glutathione for pennies on the dollar?

Surprisingly enough, this is pretty easy to do. We just need to give the body what it needs. This leads us to precursors. Precursors are the building blocks that your body needs to make glutathione. The good news is there are only three of these. Each is widely available and relatively inexpensive. The first ingredient is N-acetyl L-cysteine (NAC) which can be found in most health stores. The remaining ingredients are vitamin C and whey protein. Think of this as baking your own glutathione cake. The better the ingredients, the better the results will be. With that in mind, it's probably best to skip those "bargain" supplements sold at the big box store.

Letting your body make its own glutathione will allow it to reach its own optimal level. And once it does, a noticeable improvement in health comes to the surface. Glutathione can then reclaim its title as "the body's master antioxidant," going about its job of maintaining the balance of reduction and oxidation. Glutathione does a wonderful job of repairing proteins that have become damaged by oxidative stress. At the same time, glutathione neutralizes the current imbalances of free radicals. This helps control their damaging effects, which are often associated with premature aging.

To be clear, having sufficient glutathione in your tank can make the difference between good health and getting sick. That said, it's worth noting that glutathione cannot do all of this alone. Nope, it performs these tasks with the help of certain enzymes. Enzymes act as the catalyst that makes specific biochemical reactions happen. Without them, glutathione would be rendered ineffective.

Why is this important to know?

Well, when a substance such as mercury is attached to a cell, a family of enzymes known as glutathione S-transferases (GST) guides it into the hands of glutathione. All of this happens in Phase II detoxification. Phase II is just a step where harmful toxins are neutralized and turned into water-soluble toxins. If it helps, imagine all those tiny enzymes holding plastic spoons as they mix mercury with urine. It's an odd example I know, but sometimes odd examples help to get my point across. Once toxins become water soluble, it's easier for them to be expelled out of the body via the kidneys.

All things being equal, mercury can also be transported through the blood to the liver. It then goes from the liver into the bile, and then out to the small intestine. Who knew that urine and feces were so important?

As a side note: Insoluble fibers found in strawberries are known to capture over 95% of dietary mercury! If you eat sushi, this is good to know as (organic) strawberries reduce the amount of mercury found in contaminated fish.

Nrf2

Moving along nicely, once we have our glutathione levels topped up, we can then tackle the next part of the detox puzzle. For this, we simply need to upregulate nuclear factor erythroid 2–related factor 2, which is a key regulator of the cellular antioxidant response. *Whoa! What the heck does that mean?*

At this point, I expect I'm going to be working for my tips. Not least, because Nuclear factor erythroid 2–related factor 2 upregulation (**Nrf2 for short**) is a challenge to break down into plain English. And if I can pull this off, I'll be sure to take a bow at the end.

Ready?

At the last count, scientists estimate that the human body has around 25,000 genes in its genome. The genome is the DNA that encourages those 25,000 genes to act a certain way.

Genes are what make us who we are. And while we all share some gene characteristics (like most of us have only one head) many characteristics are unique to each of us. As an example: we all have fingers, but our fingerprints are unique to each of us.

But what has any of this got to do with detoxification or the Nrf2 pathway?

Well, fingerprints aside, those 25,000 genes tell each of your cells what to do and when to do it. This is huge as your body is mostly made up of cells, be it muscle, bone, nerve, and so on. (Phew, that last sentence saved us going off on a two-hour biology lesson).

At one time, the consensus within the medical field was that you are stuck with the genes handed to you at birth. And if some of those genes happen to be a little crappy, then there wasn't much you could do about it. Too bad, so sad. However, we now know this isn't strictly true. The way genes act is influenced by nutrients (AKA food.) Stay with me here because this next bit is incredibly relevant.

When your body needs to repair itself, certain genes are turned up. (Notice I said turned up, not on and off.) This distinction is an important one. *Here's why ...*

In your mind's eye, imagine an electric light switch being turned off and on. It's a pretty basic design for stopping and starting the flow of electricity. But there's a much fancier option for doing this. It's called a dimmer switch. Dimmer switches give us more control over how much of that light is expressed. Think of those 25,000 (ish) genes as acting in the same way. They don't turn on and off like a light switch, rather, they are being turned up and down to match the body's needs.

Here's an example of that: If we twist our ankle (always a bummer) inflammation is quickly turned all the way up. This sends out more healing nutrients to the area. As the injury heals, less inflammation is then required. But inflammation is never fully turned off, it's simply turned waaaaay down. Kinda like the dimmer switch we just mentioned.

This process is self-regulated by the immune system. But further upstream, the genes are being expressed in a way to influence the immune system. Ahh, all is clear, but how does Nrf2 fit into all of this?

I'm so glad you asked.

Nrf2 is an extremely important pathway. It's also one of the key proteins found in the body and is present in pretty much every cell. It performs a bunch of different tasks. One of those is to help upregulate the protective enzymes and protective proteins found inside the cells. Put simply, this helps the cells to protect themselves from a wide range of chronic diseases. That's a pretty neat trick, but Nrf2 is far from being a one-trick pony.

Check this out…

Whenever a stressor hits the body (like inflammation) Nrf2 springs into action. It then binds to something called the antioxidant response element. This, in turn, controls antioxidant production. At this point, our old friend glutathione is pumped around the body like it's going out of fashion. *But wait, there's more…*

Once Nrf2 gets activated, your mitochondria begin to produce more ATP. (Think of ATP as the fuel that powers the body.) *Here's where it gets interesting.*

As Nrf2 responds to oxidative stress, it takes control over 500 or so genes. To ensure the cells are protected from harmful situations, Nrf2 works with each of these genes collectively. Some genes are turned up; others are turned down. But not for too long. As we learned earlier, everything in the body needs to be balanced. Too much expression of Nrf2, over too long of a period, may even promote the development of cancerous tumors. I kid you not. But that's not the case here. With the right balance, the genes controlled by Nrf2 can be thought of as our survival genes.

And here's where this all neatly dovetails together.

Just about every illness known to man can be linked to any one of the following four things.

1: An excess of inflammation.

2: Excess toxicity.

3: A deficiency in key nutrients.

4: Too much oxidative stress which causes us to age. Nrf2 is doing all that it can to keep these things in range.

However, there are times when Nrf2 is sitting ideally on the sidelines waiting for a problem to solve. It's like having a high-powered sports car sitting in the garage. That's a shame as once Nrf2 makes more glutathione, it allows us to crank the detox handle more than normal.

Hmm, if only there was a way to somehow upregulate Nrf2. That would be like having our sweaty little fingers on all of those dimmer switches! I know what you are thinking because I had the same thought, how do we upregulate Nrf2?

That's a great question, and there are several ways to do it. First, let's start with sulforaphane.

Sulforaphane is a potent compound that kicks Nrf2 in the pants and shouts, "hey, wake up Mr. Sleepyhead, it's time to get to work."

SULFORAPHANE

The trick is to find a pure, natural source of sulforaphane. But you aren't going to find the best quality online, and you won't find it in your doctor's office. But you can find it growing in my garden. Before you beat a path to my door, see if you can guess what it is that I'm growing. If you guessed broccoli sprouts, then you would be correct.

Broccoli sprouts contain glucoraphanin which in turn creates a highly potent form of sulforaphane. If you only take one thing away from this book, then let it be the benefit of eating fresh broccoli sprouts. In case you missed it, Broccoli sprouts accelerate the body's ability to detoxify. The idea is not to go faster than your body can handle. Remember, detoxification is a marathon race, rather than a sprint.

In the interest of providing value, here are some more ways to upregulate Nrf2. The first is by adding more cruciferous veggies and sulfur-based compounds into your diet. These can be found in the allium family (onions, shallots, and garlic, etc.).

As a side note: There are lots more healing foods to be found in my book "The Healing Point."

SUPPLEMENTS

Make no mistake, broccoli sprouts are your least expensive option. But if you have a little cash to flash, you can also coax Nrf2 out of its shell with a few well-targeted supplements such as DHA, R-lipoic acid, and PQQ.

DHA is a type of omega-3 fat found in fish oils. Most people lack omega-3 fats in their diet, which causes an imbalance in the body's omega-3 to omega-6 fat ratio. DHA can help turn down inflammation, it's also pretty good for the brain and heart health. I like the brand of DHA sold by Nordic Naturals, as it's been screened (by a third party) for mercury.

R LIPOIC is significantly more potent than Alpha Lipoic Acid, hence, it's always best to **start small and go slow.** R-lipoic acid is an essential cofactor for many enzymes involved in energy production. It's of interest to us here as the body recognizes it better than Alpha Lipoic Acid.

PQQ is about 100 times as powerful as Vitamin C. It was first discovered as a cofactor for enzyme reactions in bacteria. A "cofactor," simply means it helps enzymes do their job. PQQ improves cellular energy and cognitive performance. As we age, the performance of mitochondria declines. To keep this simple, PQQ enhances the formation of new mitochondria. The downside of PQQ is some folks may find it too stimulating. The workaround for this is to take regular breaks from it. This leads us nicely into something known as "pulsing".

PULSING

Without wanting to sound like a broken record, everything within the body is a fine balance. Attempting to Upregulate Nrf2 is *not* something you want to do all day, every day.

Best results come when supplements such as R-lipoic acid are taken for a short period and then stopped. This technique is often referred to as "pulsing". Pulsing stimulates the system. It also gives the body a chance to regroup and regenerate once we do stop. It's like taking a brisk walk around the park and then pausing to sit on the park bench to catch a breath of fresh air.

Depending on your current ability to detoxify, it's important to find a sweet spot that works for you. Some folks find that "pulsing" with supplements for five days on and then taking a break for two days works best. Others may find better results from doing four days on and three days off. It depends on your tolerance for things. If at any time you feel worse, stop. Then go back to adding more binders while at the same time drinking more water.

Although supplements are a way to upregulate Nrf2, it's important to understand that you cannot supplement your way out of a poor diet. Good nutrition is the foundation of good health. And on the opposite end of the spectrum, we now find ourselves talking about fasting. When combined with exercise, fasting is yet another way to upregulate Nrf2.

FASTING

The word "fasting" conjures up all sorts of images in the mind. Let's begin with what fasting *isn't*. Fasting isn't sitting cross-legged under a tree eating twigs and berries for an extended time.

Yes, it's true, some fasts can last for days or even weeks. But most of the time, fasting is done in short bursts. This is commonly known as *intermittent* fasting. Unless you possess the rare ability to eat while you are asleep, YOU have been doing this for most of your life. Usually, until breakfast, which translates into "breaking the fast."

The idea of intermittent fasting is to prolong the window from the time we wake up to the time when we eat our first meal. In effect, we are choosing to eat within a specific time frame. This is sometimes known as the 16/8 method. For example, if your last meal is taken at 8 p.m. and you don't eat until noon the following day, then technically you have just fasted for sixteen hours straight. *That wasn't too bad, was it?*

Here's some good news. The health benefits that come with fasting go well beyond Nrf2 upregulation. During a prolonged fast, the body enters a process known as autophagy. This is where the body begins to clean out old or damaged cells. With less junk clogging up the system, things tend to run smoother. It's the equivalent of removing all those old cat videos from your cell phone.

Okay, we've covered a lot of complex issues together, and hopefully, I've given you a few things to think about and maybe even made you smile in the process. In the interest of providing value, I'd like to share one last detoxification tip with you.

INFRARED

Heat exposure activates Nrf2, heat also makes us sweat. This, in turn, allows us to shed more toxins. I like this idea as sweating lifts some of the burdens off the liver and kidneys. In case you missed it, the skin is the body's largest detoxification organ.

There are lots of ways to work up a sweat, but my favorite is to use an infrared sauna. If you don't have a sauna on hand, all is not lost. Your local gym may have one you can utilize. Often, it's included in the gym membership and no additional money is required.

If you're fortunate to have your own infrared sauna at home, then making it part of your detox routine is easy to do. The body does all the work while you sit back and chillax.

As I write this, I'm working on a new detox protocol called the Niacin flush. It includes the use of specific minerals, binders, and a supplement known as Niacin (B3.) When combined with sauna use, niacin helps to pull out older toxins stored in fat cells. If you are struggling to lose weight (and a change in diet hasn't helped) then an overload of toxins might be something that's holding you back. It's uncanny how heavy metals and mold can make a beeline for our hips. This is sometimes called "mid-life spread." Another way to look at it, the longer we are on this planet the more toxins we tend to acquire. Hence, detoxification should always be viewed as an ongoing process.

If you are serious about your health, owning an infrared sauna should be at the top of your wish list. Here's why…

Studies show that regular infrared sauna use not only reduces toxins, it also improves cardiovascular health. That's a pretty big deal when you stop to think that heart disease is the number one killer here in the US. According to the CDC, heart disease accounts for a whopping 23.1% of all registered deaths. That's more than 647,000 Americans dying every year!

An infrared sauna can also help with chronic fatigue, sleep issues, and depression. Personally, I find a thirty-minute session, followed by a hot shower, followed by a quick blast from a cold shower, helps to get the lymphatic system moving and elevates my mood for the rest of the day.

Regular infrared sauna use can also help with lingering injuries. It does this by penetrating deep into joints, muscles, and tissues. As it does so, it increases oxygen flow and circulation. This can help improve stiffness and painful joints. Infrared sauna use can even help with toxic mold exposure. The link between heavy metals and mold is an important one.

At best, mold will add to your toxic burden, at worst, it causes a bottleneck and slows down the entire detoxification process. Statistically, people with an unresolved heavy metals issue are more prone to certain molds. But wait there's more … People with an ongoing mold issue are more prone to contracting Lyme disease. *Why?*

　　Metals and mold are a drag on the immune system. An infected tick bite becomes the final straw that breaks the camel's back. The good news is once mold is dealt with the body becomes much better at managing Lyme disease.

　　Before rushing out to buy a sauna, it's important to find one with a low EMF (electric magnetic field) reading. I did quite a bit of research in this area and discovered some companies "claim" to have low EMF readings, but when you dig a little deeper, this isn't always the case. Often, isolated parts of the sauna are sent away for testing. When the results come back, the company claims that the sauna has been "independently" tested. They then slap a low EMF sticker on it, which *isn't* telling us the whole story. As with most things, you tend to get what you pay for. Cheap saunas may sound good in theory, but not if they add to your toxic burden.

　　The sauna I eventually chose came directly from the manufacturer. It arrived on my doorstep with the promise of ultra-low EMF readings. Once it was set up, I was able to replicate the company's numbers by using my own EMF meter. Seeing this with my own eyes gave me peace of mind.

As fall turns to winter, I seem to be spending more time basking in infrared rays. The heat isn't as intense as a regular sauna, it's more like the comforting heat you get from sitting by a campfire. This makes it an altogether pleasurable experience. To be clear, you'll still sweat. As you do so toxic heavy metals and PCB's etc. pour out of the skin. This takes the burden off the liver and kidneys. The trick is to use a binder that stops all those toxins from recirculating back into the system.

Details of the sauna I use can be found at the back of this book. I've also added a promo code that will save you some money.

For now, I guess that's it except to say thank *you* for spending your time with me. I hope this information has been helpful. If so, could you please help me out with a short review? **It doesn't have to be anything fancy; a simple sentence will do.** As an independent author, I rely on word of mouth for every book sale.

Last but not least, thank you to my wife and family. Without their support, writing these books would not be possible.

Until next time, bye for now.

James.

MORE BOOKS BY THIS AUTHOR

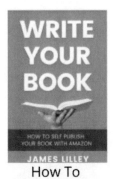
How To

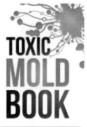
Healthy Home

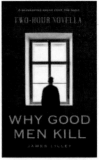
Short story

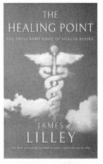
Immune Boost

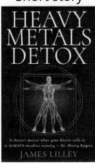
Detoxifiction

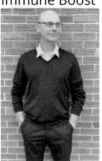
More soon

WHAT AM I UP TO NOW?

Because the liver plays such an important role in detoxification, I thought it would be helpful to dedicate an entire book to the topic. A healthy liver will allow you to heal faster, have more energy, and enjoy a peaceful state of mind. The positive effects of this can be both liberating and profound.

As always, I aim to present information in a way that's enjoyable to read. I don't think it helps anyone when a book reads like a medical dictionary. Least of all, to the person dealing with toxicity.

You can help support my efforts by signing up for my newsletter. When the book is complete, you'll be the first to know.

NEWSLETTER DETAILS

In my Fall 2020 newsletter, I attached a video where I'm sprinting against a group of teenage boys. I think they were a little confused about how an old white man (I'm almost 60) could keep up with them, lol.

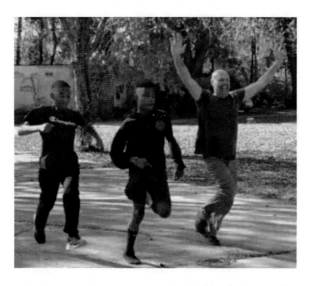

Signing up for my newsletter is free and easy to do. Rest assured, I'll never share your information and I only write when I have something of interest to say. Check it out at <u>writeonjames.com</u>

SEE YOUR NAME IN PRINT

As a hybrid author, I also enjoy writing short stories. Sometimes, I'll run fun competitions via my newsletter and the winner's name becomes a character in my next book. If you have ever wanted to see your name in print, be sure to stay in my loop.

WriteonJames.com

SAUNA DISCOUNT CODE

The low EMF sauna I'm using here is a single person unit. The company also offers two and three person units. You can save yourself a few hundred bucks by using the discount code JAMES500. Last I checked, it was good for a $500 discount.

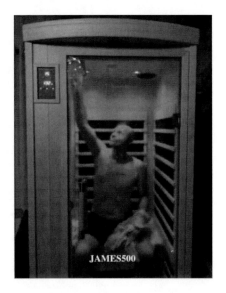

You can buy direct from the manufacturer at radianthealthsaunas.com. Or, if you need help ordering this sauna you can shoot me an email at Jameslilley24@gmail.com Just add the word SAUNA in the subject line.

NOTES